AN ILLUSTRAT

Gastr_____gy

Commissioning Editor: Laurence Hunter
Project Development Managers: Jim Killgore and Lynn Watt
Project Manager: Nancy Arnott
Designer: Sarah Russell
Page Layout: Archetype Graphic Communication, Peebles

AN ILLUSTRATED COLOUR TEXT

Gastroenterology

Graham P. Butcher

Consultant Physician and Gastroenterologist
Southport District General Hospital, UK

Illustrated by Robert Britton

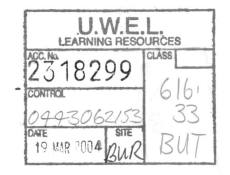
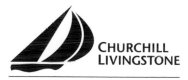

CHURCHILL LIVINGSTONE

EDINBURGH LONDON NEW YORK PHILADELPHIA ST LOUIS SYDNEY TORONTO 2003

CHURCHILL LIVINGSTONE
An imprint of Elsevier Science Limited

First published 2003

ISBN 0443 06215 3

British Library Cataloguing in Publication Data
A catalogue record for this book is available from the British Library

Library of Congress Cataloging in Publication Data
A catalog record for this book is available from the Library of Congress

Note
Medical knowledge is constantly changing. As new information becomes available, changes in treatment, procedures, equipment and the use of drugs become necessary. The authors and the publishers have taken care to ensure that the information given in this text is accurate and up to date. However, readers are strongly advised to confirm that the information, especially with regard to drug usage, complies with the latest legislation and standards of practice.

 your source for books, journals and multimedia in the health sciences
www.elsevierhealth.com

The
publisher's
policy is to use
**paper manufactured
from sustainable forests**

Printed in China

PREFACE

The object of this book is to approach gastroenterology in the way that patients present, rather than in traditional organ based physiology and pathology. Both approaches have drawbacks, and diseases do not necessarily fit cleanly into either grouping. We have attempted to cover topics in two-page 'learning units' but of necessity some require more extensive coverage and this has been given. In keeping with other books in this series, the format uses individually designed double page spreads, generously illustrated with photographs, line drawings and tables.

Summary boxes reinforce important concepts and act as revision aids.

The text is aimed at medical students, junior hospital doctors, general practitioners and specialist nurse practitioners in gastroenterology. The text labours the importance of the history and examination in clinical practice because, despite huge advances in investigations and particularly in imaging, these are the cornerstone to effective management.

G.P.B

ACKNOWLEDGEMENTS

I am indebted to my colleagues at Southport Hospital for help in preparing text and figures: Mr Mike Zciderman for the sections on surgery; Dr Steve Dundas for pathology; and Dr Peter Hughes for radiology images. I am grateful to Dr Howard Smart for reading and checking the text.

The book is dedicated to Deborah, Rhiannon and Verity.

G.P.B

CONTENTS

HISTORY

The object of this text is to approach illnesses in the way in which they present, not as ready diagnoses but rather as a complex of clinical symptoms with which patients may suffer. Consequently, some illnesses could appear in any one of a number of sections but are placed at the site which seems appropriate for their common presentation.

Gastroenterology, perhaps more than any other specialty, has to approach the patient as a whole and not as isolated systems. Many gastrointestinal (GI) illnesses have extra-intestinal or extra-hepatic manifestations affecting the nervous system, skin or joints. Conversely, many non-GI conditions, such as thyroid, adrenal and cardiovascular diseases, may present with symptoms referable to the GI tract.

This underlines the importance of a systematic history and clinical examination prior to investigation.

HISTORY OF THE PRESENTING COMPLAINT

Occasionally, abnormalities are picked up on routine screening, such as anaemia or abnormal liver function tests, but usually patients are symptomatic and present with a common range of symptoms.

DYSPHAGIA

The usual description is of food sticking or lodging at any site between the mouth and abdomen. It is helpful to determine the level at which food sticks, the duration of the symptoms and also whether it has progressed and over what timescale. Previous symptoms of gastro-oesophageal reflux suggest a peptic lesion whilst relentless progression and weight loss point to a malignant cause.

ABDOMINAL PAIN

The routine approach to any pain should be followed, with site, quality, duration, behaviour (exacerbating or relieving factors) determined. An acute presentation of abdominal pain is often due to a perforated or inflamed organ or an intra-abdominal vascular cause. The effect of food and defaecation should be elicited for more chronic abdominal pain, whilst a relationship to the menstrual cycle points to a

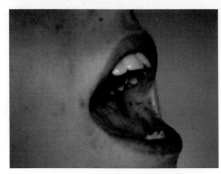

Fig. 1 **Buccal pigmentation of Peutz-Jeghers syndrome.**

gynaecological cause. There are often associated symptoms of abdominal bloating and a change in bowel habit which accompanies abdominal pain and these require specific inquiry.

CHANGE IN BOWEL HABIT

Constipation/diarrhoea

The accepted normal range of stool frequency is between three times a day and once every three days. Patients are often embarrassed to discuss their bowel habit, and it is important to put them at their ease. It is insufficient to accept descriptions of either constipation or diarrhoea alone. The frequency and consistency of the stool should be determined, and prompting may be helpful, with descriptions such as 'watery', 'porridge-like', and 'hard' or 'pellety' (like rabbit droppings). Nocturnal defaecation and urgency are important symptoms and should be enquired about specifically. Pale colour and the presence of oil suggest malabsorption. Blood in the stool can be either mixed in, suggesting a higher colonic lesion, or seen discolouring the toilet water, which suggests a lower colonic cause.

GI BLEEDING / ANAEMIA

Iron deficiency anaemia can be caused by either chronic GI blood loss, insufficient dietary intake or malabsorption of ingested iron. Blood loss may be noticed in the stool; or there may be a darkening of the stool, however it is usually unnoticed. Specific inquiry should be made regarding dietary intake of iron, particularly red meat, and evidence of malabsorption.

Acute GI bleeding usually results in haematemesis, melaena or frank PR (per rectum) bleeding accompanied by cardiovascular collapse when sufficiently large.

JAUNDICE / ABNORMAL LIVER FUNCTION TESTS

When taking a history from a jaundiced patient it is important to first determine whether the jaundice is due to cholestasis/obstruction or not. Itch, pale stools and dark urine are characteristic features of this. Specific questioning should include recent foreign travel, prescribed medication within the last 6 months, any other non-prescribed therapies or illegal drugs taken ever, with particular reference to intravenous drugs. Previous blood transfusions, episodes of jaundice or recent contact with jaundiced patients and sexual contact (particularly homosexual) should also be elicited. Family history or other illnesses within the family may be important, and particular reference should be made to alcohol consumption, documenting daily or weekly consumption.

WEIGHT LOSS

The importance of the history when dealing with a patient with weight loss cannot be overemphasised. Intake, absorption and metabolism should be considered. Is a patient eating enough to maintain an adequate weight, or is there evidence of an eating disorder or other psychological illness such as depression? Recent onset of abdominal pain or a change in the nature of previous pain should alert the clinician, whilst passage of pale stools with oil in them (steatorrhoea) suggests malabsorption, and a change in bowel habit with blood in the stools points to a colonic cause. A complete review of all systems is essential, as respiratory, cardiovascular and endocrine causes of weight loss can lead to GI symptoms causing presentation.

PAST MEDICAL HISTORY

The nature of previous surgery is often poorly understood by patients, but attempts should be made to determine what has been done previously and why. There may be a recurrence of the previous problem or a longer-term complication of the surgery. If there is access to previous medical notes then it may be helpful to know whether abnormalities in blood tests (such as liver function tests) have been long standing.

FAMILY HISTORY

This is obviously relevant for directly inherited disorders (Table 1 and Fig. 1) but is also important for polygenic illnesses, such as colitis, colon cancer and coeliac disease, where having affected relatives increases a patient's risk of developing that condition. Inquiry into where the family has come from may be helpful, as certain conditions are more prevalent in various parts of the world, such as coeliac disease in southern Ireland and intestinal tuberculosis in developing countries.

Knowledge of the mode of inheritance and relative risks will help in counselling both patients and their families.

SOCIAL HISTORY

Smoking habit, alcohol consumption and employment may all help to reach a diagnosis, but many GI conditions are chronic and a good knowledge of domestic circumstances, family life and hopes and expectations will facilitate managing a patient long-term.

ALLERGIES

On a general note, patients often have misconceptions regarding true drug allergies. If a patient suggests they are allergic to an antibiotic, the exact circumstances of what occurred should be clarified (e.g. did they develop a rash?). Dietary intolerances are often perceived as allergies and, again, clarification in the history is required.

DRUG HISTORY

Many drugs may affect the GI tract – not only drugs currently being taken but those taken months previously (Fig. 2). All drugs should be treated with suspicion, but the commonest offenders are listed (Table 2). If there is doubt regarding a drug, authoritative texts or the manufacturers should be consulted.

REVIEW OF SYSTEMS

It is quicker to run through all the systems the first time a patient is interviewed than to realise a relevant piece of information was missed after several fruitless investigations.

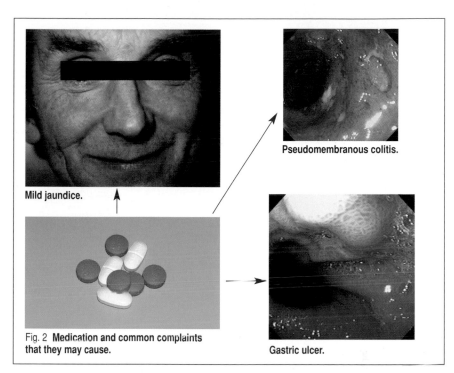

Mild jaundice.

Pseudomembranous colitis.

Gastric ulcer.

Fig. 2 **Medication and common complaints that they may cause.**

Table 1 **Some of the directly inherited diseases that can affect the gastrointestinal tract**

Diseases	Inheritance	Characteristics
Liver		
Wilson's disease	AR	Increased copper deposition in liver and brain
Haemochromatosis	AR	Increased iron deposition in liver, skin, pancreas
Oesophagus		
Tylosis	AD	Hyperkeratosis of hands and squamous cell carcinoma of the oesophagus
Small bowel		
Peutz–Jeghers syndrome	AD	Pigmentation of buccal mucosa with hamartomatous polyps in small bowel and elsewhere in GI tract (Fig. 1)
Colon		
Familial adult polyposis	AD	Colonic polyps with high risk of malignant development
Hereditary non-polyposis colon cancer	AD	Colorectal cancers in colonic adenomas, without polyposis
AR = Autosomal recessive; AD = Autosomal dominant		

Table 2 **A few of the more common adverse effects caused by drugs in the GI tract**

Site	Drug	Effect
Oesophagus	Antibiotics	Candidiasis
	Potassium slow release	Mucosal ulceration
Stomach/duodenum	NSAIDs	Gastritis/duodenitis
		Ulceration/haemorrhage
Small bowel	NSAIDs	Ulceration/haemorrhage
Colon	Antibiotics	Pseudomembranous colitis
	NSAIDs	Colitis
	Iron	Constipation
Liver	Antibiotics	Cholestasis/hepatitis
	Paracetamol	Hepatitis

History

- A thorough history is essential in GI medicine as many gastroenterological conditions have systemic effects and vice versa.
- Tease out what patients mean by their descriptive terms such as 'constipation' or 'diarrhoea'.
- Social circumstances are particularly important in managing patients with chronic conditions well.
- Current medication and therapies taken within the last 6 months must be established and primary physicians should be contacted if necessary. Non-prescribed medication and drugs taken should also be determined.

EXAMINATION

Examination of the patient begins as he or she enters the consulting room, and continues whilst taking the history. This is also true when clerking a patient in the accident and emergency department – much can be gained from the way the history is given and the posture adopted.

Following the examination there may be obvious pointers to direct further investigations, such as a mass, lymph node or an enlarged liver. However, there are often no such clues and this simply emphasises the importance of a good history.

It is hopefully clear that a complete physical examination is the ideal, but it is not possible to describe this here and the reader is referred to other texts. The following will outline a scheme for examination of the GI tract.

GENERAL INSPECTION

The presence of pallor or jaundice should be noted and the patient's general demeanour observed. Difficulty with breathing or speech and concentration should be obvious, and abnormal posture, such as that due to a hemiparesis, should be noted. Skin should be inspected for rashes, such as erythema nodosum, pyoderma gangrenosum (Fig. 1) and dermatitis herpetiformis, and joints should be examined for arthropathy.

HANDS

Look for finger clubbing (Fig. 2), leuconychia, koilonychia, and Dupuytren's contracture and palmar erythema in the palms. Patients should be requested to outstretch their arms and cock their wrists back to check for a course flapping tremor as seen in hepatic encephalopathy. Pulse and blood pressure must be measured.

NECK AND HEAD

The neck should be examined for jugular venous engorgement, a goitre and lymphadenopathy. Mucous membranes in the mouth should be noted for anaemia, pigmentation, aphthous ulceration and *Candida*; the tongue for glossitis and telangectasia; the teeth for damage and lips for angular stomatitis.

CHEST WALL

This should be inspected for spider naevi and (in men) the presence of gynaecomastia.

ABDOMEN

Inspect for distension and previous surgical scars, and note distended veins – if emanating and filling from the umbilicus this indicates portal venous obstruction (caput medusae). Employ light palpation for tenderness, rigidity or guarding, observing the patient's face whilst examining, followed by firmer palpation for masses (Table 1) and then specific examination for enlarged liver, spleen and kidneys. If the liver is enlarged (Fig. 3) its size and consistency should be determined and particularly careful examination for the spleen performed (Table 2). Percussion of the upper

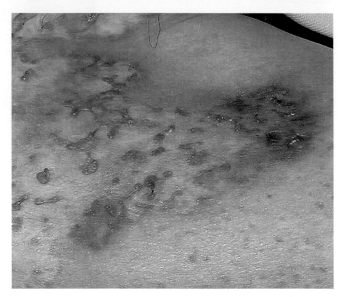

Fig. 1 **Pyoderma gangrenosum.**

border of the liver is important to determine its upper margin, which should be in the fifth intercostal space. It may be displaced downwards by a low diaphragm, as in emphysema, which will give the impression of an enlarged liver if only the abdomen is examined. Percussion is the only technique which will clinically demonstrate a shrunken liver, as seen in cirrhosis.

Examine for shifting dullness or fluid thrill for ascites. Auscultate for the quantity and characteristics of the bowel sounds.

Anal examination for haemorrhoids, mucosal prolapse, tumours and fistulae should precede rectal examination which examines both the mucosa and faeces – these should be inspected for colour and consistency on the glove.

Table 1 **Differential diagnosis of masses in the right iliac fossa and the epigastrium**

Right iliac fossa	Epigastrium
Caecal mass – tumour or faeces	Gastric tumour
Terminal ileal thickening (Crohn's/TB)	Pancreatic tumour or cyst
Appendix mass	Abdominal aortic aneurysm
Abscess	Transverse colon tumour
Ovarian tumour	Abdominal wall mass
Abdominal wall mass	
Amoebiasis	
Intussusception	

Table 2 **Causes of hepatomegaly**

Fatty liver – smooth and firm
Hepatic tumour (primary or secondaries) – hard and irregular
Right ventricular failure – firm and smooth, possibly pulsatile
Hepatic vein thrombosis (Budd-Chiari) – firm, smooth and tender
Myeloproliferative disorders – smooth and firm
Infective (viral, abscesses, hydatid cyst)
Storage disorders (amyloidosis, Gaucher's, haemochromatosis)

With splenomegaly
Infective – infectious mononucleosis
Myeloproliferative – myelofibrosis, chronic myeloid leukaemia
Portal hypertension – when associated with hepatomegaly
Reticuloses
Storage disorders (Gaucher's, amyloidosis)
Anaemia (pernicious anaemia)

Sigmoidoscopy

This is usually only helpful when the rectum is empty. It allows direct inspection of the rectal mucosa for the presence of colitis and also allows mucosal or lesion biopsy (Fig. 4). However, the view is often obscured by faeces and subsequent flexible sigmoidoscopic examination should be performed following an enema.

CLINICAL GROUPINGS

The experienced clinician seeks out certain combinations of signs rather than simply examining for all possibilities. Examples include:

- *Stigmata of chronic liver disease* (in the jaundiced patient) which include Dupuytren's contracture, gynaecomastia, spider naevi and signs of portal hypertension which would be unusual in an acute liver disease.
- *Portal hypertension* is suggested by splenomegaly, ascites and caput medusae.
- *Hepatic encephalopathy* is suggested by a slow flapping tremor, foetor hepaticus and constructional apraxia.
- *Inflammatory bowel disease* is suggested by oral ulceration, skin rashes (pyoderma gangrenosum or erythema nodosum), arthritis and iritis.
- *Primary biliary cirrhosis* is suggested by jaundice, xanthelasma and skin excoriation.
- *Eating disorders* are suggested by wasting, lanugo, abnormal dentition associated with repeated vomiting and thickened skin on the dorsum of the fingers caused by repeated self-induced vomiting.

EPONYMOUS SIGNS AND 'LAWS'

One way that medicine honours its finest practitioners has been to name signs or diseases after those that described them. This is becoming less popular but here are some that are still in usage:

- **Murphy's sign.** Pain on deep inspiration whilst the examining hand is placed below the right costal margin is a positive sign and suggests inflammatory gallbladder disease.
- **Grey Turner's sign.** Extravasation of blood from haemorrhagic pancreatitis to produce discoloration in the flanks or around the umbilicus (**Cullen's sign**).
- **Troisier's sign.** Palpable lymph node in the left supraclavicular fossa (Virchow's node) associated with metastatic gastric cancer.
- **Courvoisier's law.** A palpable gallbladder in the presence of jaundice suggests that the jaundice is unlikely to be due to gallstones and pancreatic cancer is more likely (Mirizzi's

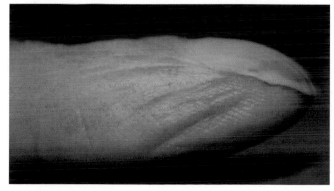

Fig. 2 **Finger clubbing.**

syndrome – an impacted stone in the cystic duct causing partial obstruction of the common hepatic duct – is one exception).

INVESTIGATION

Each section in this book features an investigation algorithm. These help to formulate an investigation plan but cannot be all inclusive. They are led by a good history and examination, and results should always be interpreted in this light.

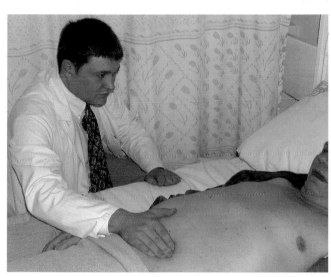

Fig. 3 **Examination of the abdomen.**

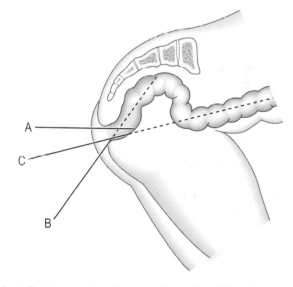

Fig. 4 **Technique of sigmoidoscopy.** Initial insertion (**A**) through anus. Advance to **B** and then straighten sigmoid colon by advancing to position **C**.

Examination

- Inspection of the patient should begin when they are first met and continue until the end of the clerking.
- A full general examination is the ideal.
- Do not ignore clinical signs that you may imagine do not fit your diagnosis. Always keep an open mind.
- If you elicit one sign of chronic liver disease, specifically search for others; likewise with portal hypertension, heart failure, malabsorption, eating disorder, etc.

STANDARD INVESTIGATIONS I

ENDOSCOPY

Gastroscopy (oesophago-gastro-duodenoscopy / OGD) (Fig. 1)

Indications

OGD is usually the first investigation for dysphagia, odynophagia, dyspepsia, gastro-oesophageal reflux and recurrent vomiting. The procedure also allows interventions such as biopsy, dilatation of strictures, insertion of prostheses for palliation of malignant strictures, injection therapy for bleeding lesions and placement of gastrostomy tubes.

Technique

All endoscopes are essentially similar with a flexible distal tip which is controlled by two wheels allowing right, left, up and down movements. There is an operating or biopsy channel, and a separate channel which passes air to distend the organ under examination. Water can also be passed down this channel to wash the lens. Suction can be applied via the operating channel. Air/water and suction are controlled by blue and red buttons on the control head (Fig. 2).

Following a period of fasting (4–6 hours), patients are placed on their left side and the oropharynx is anaesthetised by topical anaesthetic. The patient may or may not be sedated, depending upon preference. Patient care during the procedure requires maintenance of the airway and adequate oxygenation.

Intubation of the oesophagus is usually undertaken under direct vision, and then the oesophagus, stomach and the duodenum to the third part are inspected. Careful attention is paid to areas that are difficult to see, such as the gastric fundus, which is best seen by retroverting ('J'ing) the gastroscope.

Sedation. The usual sedative is an intravenous short-acting benzodiazepine such as midazolam, which has both sedating and amnesic effects. The principal risk of sedation is suppression of breathing, and training is essential to allow the clinician to correctly titrate doses – for midazolam doses range from 2 mg for an elderly frail women or child to 10 mg or occasionally more in a large man who may be currently using a benzodiazepine.

The benzodiazepine receptor antagonist flumazenil allows rapid reversal of the

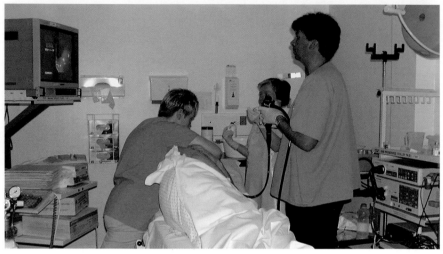

Fig. 1 **Gastroscopy.**

effects of benzodiazepines, and should always be immediately to hand for emergency use. Its effects take less than a minute, and it should be used when oversedation has occurred and breathing has been suppressed.

Opiate analgesia, such as pethidine, is used for potentially painful procedures such as colonoscopy or ERCP; however, opiates compound the effects of benzodiazepines and their dose should therefore be reduced, by approximately 50%. Venous access is best achieved with a cannula in the right hand, as patients lie on their left and in so doing may impede venous drainage on that side. The cannula should only be removed when the patient is fully awake.

Topical anaesthesia (lignocaine throat spray) is usually used to aid intubation by reducing gagging. Patients should not be allowed to drink until topical anaesthesia has worn off and should not drive or operate machinery for 24 hours following sedation.

If a procedure has been undertaken that has the potential to perforate the oesophagus, patients should be examined for surgical emphysema, a chest X-ray can be performed, and if symptoms or signs are suggestive, a gastrografin swallow should also be carried out.

Potential complications

- Those related to sedation.
- Aspiration.
- Those related to specific procedures, such as perforation or haemorrhage.

Obtain signed, informed consent by explaining the procedure, the possibility of

sore throat following it, and risks associated with planned interventions.

Flexible sigmoidoscopy

Indications

The flexible sigmoidoscope is used in the investigation of rectal bleeding, rectal pain, change in bowel habit and screening for colorectal cancer. It allows monitoring of ulcerative colitis, and should be performed whenever a barium enema is requested.

Technique

Flexible sigmoidoscopy is often performed without sedation. The patient's lower bowel is prepared with an enema and the patient is placed on his or her left side. The sigmoidoscope is introduced into the rectum following a digital examination of the anorectal canal – performed to avoid missing lesions of the anal canal, which may not be well visualised during the procedure. A view is usually obtained to the splenic flexure.

Potential complications

- Those related to sedation
- Those related to specific procedures, such as perforation or haemorrhage.

Obtain signed, informed consent by explaining the procedure, indicating that if a polyp is seen this may be removed at the time. Explain that there is a very low risk of perforating the bowel, particularly if a polypectomy is performed, and that haemorrhage may occur if a biopsy or polypectomy is undertaken, but that this usually stops spontaneously.

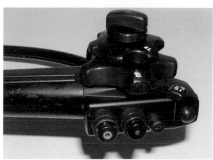

Fig. 2 **Control head of colonoscope showing wheels for steering, and buttons for air/water and suction.**

Colonoscopy

Indications

Colonoscopy is indicated for:

* investigation of iron deficiency anaemia
* follow-up of abnormal barium enema
* investigation of change in bowel habit
* colorectal cancer screening
* staging and surveillance in ulcerative colitis.

It also allows procedures such as polypectomy, or stent insertion.

Technique

The bowel is prepared by cleansing with a strong stimulant laxative such as picolax or an osmotic laxative such as polyethylene glycol solution, which is taken the day prior to the investigation. Iron is discontinued several days earlier and warfarin replaced with heparin if polypectomy is to be carried out. The patient is asked to give consent and receives sedation and analgesia. Colonoscopy follows digital examination of the anorectal canal and a complete colonoscopy is one that reaches the caecum, or better still the terminal ileum (small bowel biopsies confirm complete colonic examination). Poor bowel preparation, looping of the colonoscope and patient discomfort may be reasons for an incomplete examination. It is essential that the colonoscopist recognises when an incomplete examination has been performed, so that further imaging may be undertaken, such as a barium enema. A major potential hazard is an unrecognised incomplete examination, which has the potential of missing proximal lesions. After the procedure, patients have some gaseous abdominal distension which soon passes.

Potential complications

These are the same as for flexible sigmoidoscopy, but the risk of perforation is higher, particularly if right sided colonic polyps are removed.

Endoscopic retrograde cholangiopancreatography (ERCP)

Indications

Diagnostic ERCP is becoming less common as better imaging techniques such as ultrasound and CT allow the endoscopist to know what to expect during the procedure. Investigation and treatment of obstructive jaundice, cholangitis and pancreatitis are the most usual indications.

Technique

Preparation of the patient is as for gastroscopy with the usual addition of analgesia. A platelet count and clotting tests are performed and anomalies are corrected prior to the procedure. Blood is grouped and saved. A side-viewing endoscope is used (Fig. 3) to allow a view of the papilla, which is cannulated with a cannula filled with X-ray contrast medium. This allows accurate localisation and diagnosis. Sphincterotomy, stent insertion, and stone crushing or removal are all possible during the procedure. Particularly when there is an obstructed biliary system, antibiotic prophylaxis is given prior to the procedure and for a few days afterwards. Ciprofloxacin is a good choice for this.

Potential complications

* Those related to sedation.
* Following sphincterotomy, haemorrhage may occur in up to 10% of cases and is usually treated with injection at the site with adrenaline. Rarely, surgical intervention is required if bleeding continues.
* Perforation of bowel or bile duct may occur following sphincterotomy or cannulation. If biliary drainage into the bowel is established and maintained, it is usual for leaks to close spontaneously.
* Pancreatitis occurs in approximately 10% of cases and is recognised by abdominal pain and a rise in the serum amylase following the procedure.

Serious pancreatitis occurs in around 1% and carries a recognised mortality. This is the most major complication and patients must be made fully aware of this eventuality prior to giving consent.

Obtain signed, informed consent by explaining the procedure, particularly highlighting the specific potential complications outlined above.

Enteroscopy

Indications

Enteroscopy is indicated for obscure gastrointestinal bleeding, particularly related to NSAID usage, and assessment of small bowel diseases such as Crohn's disease.

Technique

Following bowel preparation an overtube is used with the long flexible enteroscope, so that the portion of the enteroscope passing through the stomach and into the duodenum can be stiffened to prevent intragastric looping. This allows introduction into the distal small bowel. The full circumference of the bowel may not be visualised and small lesions such as angiodysplasia may be missed.

Potential complications

* Those related to sedation.
* Damage to the upper gastrointestinal tract, with tears and perforations, caused by the overtube.

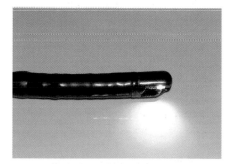

Fig. 3 **Side-viewing duodenoscope for ERCP.**

Standard investigations I

* Always take time to explain the planned procedure.
* Have a thorough understanding of the procedure and its potential complications.
* Do not be afraid to tell patients of potential hazards. It is up to them if they are willing to undertake the procedure.
* If patients have discomfort or pain after a procedure consider potential complications.

STANDARD INVESTIGATIONS II

RADIOLOGY

Barium swallow with fluoroscopy

This is a technique which allows evaluation of the swallowing mechanism and can determine if aspiration is recurring, particularly after strokes. It is also useful in evaluating pharyngeal pouches.

Barium meal

Largely superseded by gastroscopy, this has the benefit of being performed without sedation and may be useful when patients have dysphagia with a normal gastroscopy. It is useful for detecting motility problems.

Barium follow-through

This is used to image the small bowel. The patient takes the contrast orally, but views of the terminal ileum may be poor and strictures may be missed.

Small bowel enema

This allows better imaging of the small bowel than a barium follow-through but has the disadvantage that small bowel intubation is required, which patients find uncomfortable. Small bowel strictures and the terminal ileum are better seen than with barium follow-through (Fig. 1).

Barium enema

This is a widely practised procedure (Fig. 2) which allows rapid imaging of the colon following bowel preparation. Safer and quicker to perform than colonoscopy, and requiring no sedation or analgesia, it allows detection of mucosal lesions down to 1 cm. It may also give information about mucosal irregularity such as in inflammatory bowel disease, but should not be performed if active disease is present. The procedure gives no information about lesions such as angiodysplasia.

Defaecating proctogram

X-ray contrast is mixed with a thickening agent to simulate faeces and is introduced into the rectum. The patient is asked to expel this material whilst X-ray images are obtained. This technique can be useful in obstructed defaecation and in the rectal prolapse syndrome.

Colonic transit studies

These allow assessment of patients who complain of constipation, particularly those who claim to open their bowels very infrequently. Radio-opaque markers are taken orally and their position confirmed by a straight abdominal X-ray. X-rays are taken over subsequent days and the pellets remaining are counted. Normal ranges are available depending upon the particular protocol followed.

ULTRASOUND

This is a widely used technique to view the liver, gallbladder, biliary tree and spleen. It is also very helpful in assessing masses to determine their nature – solid or cystic. The technique is particularly prone to user interpretation, as the images produced are not easy for secondary analysis. It is frequently used to guide the radiologist in targeting biopsies, and is quick and non-invasive with no significant risk or discomfort to the patient.

Endoscopic ultrasound has the ultrasound probe at the distal end of the endoscope and allows assessment of mucosal lesions, such as early cancers in the oesophagus or stomach. Experienced practitioners can detect transmural spread and local lymph nodes.

COMPUTERISED TOMOGRAPHY

This technique allows detection of some lesions down to 1 cm and is particularly useful in assessing the liver for mass lesions and detecting local and more distant spread of tumours. CT imaging is most useful in visualising the pancreas, as overlying bowel gas can impair the view obtained at ultrasound.

MAGNETIC RESONANCE IMAGING

This technique is becoming increasingly useful at visualising the biliary tree to detect stones, which are often not well seen by either ultrasound or CT. It is non-invasive and without irradiation to the patient, and can also be used in the pelvis for outlining routes of fistulae.

ISOTOPE SCANNING

Labelled white cell scan

White blood cells are removed and labelled with either technetium or indium and reintroduced into the patient. White cell migration occurs to areas of inflammation allowing areas of colitis or ileitis to be demonstrated. The technique may also be useful for detecting abscesses.

HIDA scan

This depends on a technetium-labelled isotope being selectively taken up by the liver and excreted into the bile. It demonstrates a non-filling gallbladder in acute cholecystitis with an otherwise patent biliary system, and may be useful in those with acalculous biliary pain and in demonstrating delayed excretion into the duodenum in sphincter of Oddi dysfunction.

OESOPHAGEAL STUDIES

pH and manometry (Fig. 3)

Following an overnight fast, a catheter is introduced via the nose and placed within the oesophagus and stomach. Pressure transducers allow detection of peristaltic waves within the oesophagus and assess-

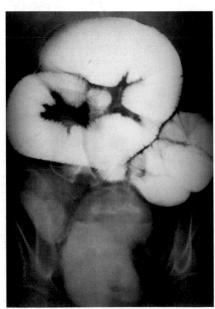

Fig. 1 **Small bowel enema showing bowel distension due to obstruction.**

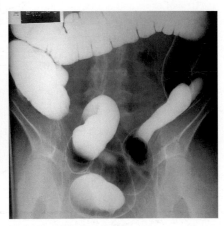

Fig. 2 **Normal barium enema.**

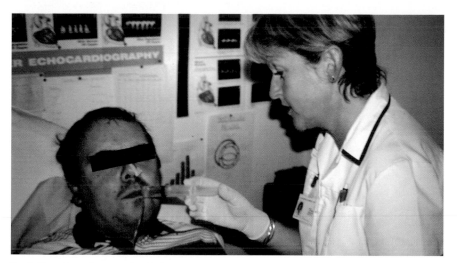

Fig. 3 **Oesophageal manometry studies.**

ment of the lower oesophageal sphincter. This method can be used to demonstrate abnormal peristalsis, achalasia and other disorders of motility. Following manometric detection of the lower oesophageal sphincter, a pH probe is placed proximal to this and left in situ for 24 hours whilst connected to a small computer, and the pH is monitored during this period. This allows quantification of gastro-oesophageal acid reflux.

BREATH TESTS

Urea breath test for *Helicobacter pylori* with ¹³C

This procedure, the most sensitive way of detecting *H. pylori*, is performed following an overnight fast. Patients are given a drink to delay gastric emptying followed by the labelled urea solution. Urease in the bacteria splits the urea to produce labelled carbon dioxide. Patients exhale into a receptacle to allow quantification.

Lactose breath test (Fig. 4)

This test is used to detect lactose intolerance (lactase deficiency). Following an overnight fast, patients are given a lactose solution and exhaled hydrogen is quantified. Lactose is usually completely absorbed in the small bowel but in the presence of lactase deficiency this does not occur and lactose reaches the colon where bacteria metabolise it, producing hydrogen. This is then measured in exhaled air.

Glucose breath test

This is a similar technique to the lactose breath test, except glucose is the carbohydrate. The procedure allows detection of small bowel bacterial overgrowth, as organisms present in the small bowel metabolise the carbohydrate prior to its complete absorption and this leads to an early rise in exhaled hydrogen.

PANCREATIC FUNCTION TESTS

Intubation tests

The duodenum is intubated so that pancreatic enzymes and bicarbonate can be aspirated and assayed. Pancreatic secretion is stimulated by cholecystokinin (CCK) and secretin. This is probably the most accurate way of assessing exocrine pancreatic function, but is a complex procedure that is not widely used in clinical practice.

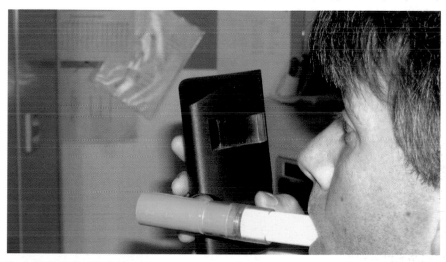

Fig. 4 **Hydrogen breath testing.**

Pancreolauryl test

Fluorescein dilaurate is given by mouth and subsequently cleaved by pancreatic esterases to produce water-soluble fluorescein. This is excreted in the urine and collected. The procedure is repeated after a few days with free fluorescein and the recovery rate expressed as a ratio. The test is useful in confirming significant pancreatic exocrine dysfunction.

NBT-PABA test (*N*-benzoyl-L-tyrosyl-para-amino benzoic acid)

NBT-PABA is cleaved by pancreatic chymotrypsin and PABA measured in serum or urine. There are dietary components and drugs that can interfere with the test's accuracy and, like the pancreolauryl test, it is most accurate when severe disease is present.

Faecal fat

There has to be a 90% reduction in pancreatic lipase excretion for steatorrhoea to develop. Faecal fat is normally less than 8%. Because of the degree of pancreatic damage that has to have occurred for steatorrhoea to develop, it is an insensitive test for the detection of pancreatic dysfunction.

Standard investigations II

- Investigation must always be preceded by a good history.
- Have a hypothesis (differential diagnosis) that your investigation will help to prove or disprove.
- Indiscriminate use of investigations will produce uninterpretable results which may prompt further inappropriate investigation.
- When in doubt, discuss with radiologists to select the most appropriate imaging.

THE CLINICAL APPROACH

HISTORY

The first thing to do when a patient describes difficulty with swallowing is establish exactly what they mean. Does he or she have difficulty initiating swallowing, or is there a sensation of food sticking between the mouth and stomach?

Difficulty initiating a swallow suggests a psychological or neurological cause. If related to anxiety (globus sensation) there may be other associated features: the patient is often young and describes the feeling of a lump in the throat, and the problem may be long- standing but intermittent. With a neurological cause there may have been a sudden onset with dysphasia, or peripheral neurological deficit when caused by a stroke (Fig. 1) or more progressive difficulties such as those associated with Parkinson's disease, motor neurone disease or myasthenia gravis.

When there is a feeling of food lodging within the oesophagus, progression should be determined: fluids are easiest to swallow whilst meat and bread are the most difficult solids. Long-standing previous reflux symptoms may suggest the development of a peptic stricture, but this has become much less frequent with the advent of effective acid suppression therapy (H_2 receptor antagonists and more recently proton pump inhibitors). Progressive dysphagia is more frequently caused by oesophageal cancer. This is usually found in the older age group, is relentlessly progressive and invariably associated with weight loss. Less common oesophageal causes include achalasia, oesophageal webs, oesophagitis, systemic sclerosis and external compression of the oesophagus by bronchial tumour, lymph nodes, aortic aneurysms and an enlarged left atrium (Table 1).

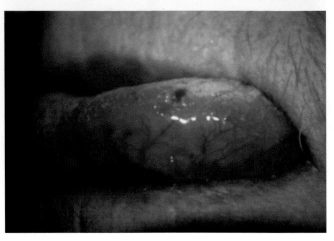

Fig. 2 **Oral telangiectasia.**

EXAMINATION

Evidence of metastatic spread from oesophageal cancers, with lymph-adenopathy in the supraclavicular fossa, should be sought. Neurological complexes associated with stroke, motor neurone disease, myasthenia gravis and Parkinson's disease should be examined for and are usually clinically obvious if advanced enough to cause swallowing difficulty. Calcinosis, telangiectasia and Raynaud's disease with systemic sclerosis indicate the CREST syndrome which is rare but frequently complicated by dysphagia (Figs 2 and 3).

INVESTIGATION

It should be obvious at the end of the history and examination whether neurological investigation should be the first step (Fig. 4). Radiology of the upper GI tract is much less frequently per-

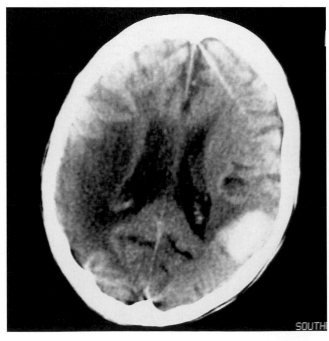

Fig. 1 **CT scan brain with haemorrhagic infarct shows as a white area in the cortex.**

Table 1 **Causes of dysphagia**

Causes	Clinical features
Common	
Carcinoma of the oesophagus	Progressive, weight loss, elderly
Peptic stricture	Previous reflux symptoms, bolus impaction
Oesophagitis	Reflux symptoms
Bulbar/pseudobulbar palsy (previous CVA)	Sudden onset, dysphasia and hemiparesis
Less common	
Achalasia	Non-acidic regurgitation, 'normal' OGD
Cricopharyngeal dysfunction	Elderly, frail, difficulty initiating swallow
External compression	Bronchial carcinoma, pharyngeal pouch, mediastinal lymph nodes, cervical spine osteophytes, aortic aneurysms
Globus sensation	Sensation of lump in throat, with difficulty initiating swallow
Diffuse oesophageal spasm	Uncoordinated, non-propulsive peristalsis
Schatzki ring	Small, distal, benign oesophageal web, bolus impaction
Postcricoid web	Iron deficiency, web, glossitis and koilonychia (Plummer–Vinson syndrome)
Systemic sclerosis (CREST)	Calcinosis in the skin, Raynaud's phenomenon, oesophageal dysfunction, sclerodactyly and telangiectasia
Decreased saliva	Drugs (anticholinergics)
Parkinson's disease	Tremor, bradykinesia and rigidity
Motor neurone disease	Muscle weakness, wasting and fasciculation
Polymyositis	Generalised progressive muscle wasting
Chagas, disease	Ganglion cell destruction by *Trypanosoma cruzi*, endemic in South America; resembles achalasia

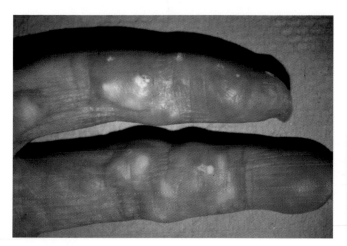

Fig. 3 **Calcinosis.**

and easier to perform and analyse with solid state technology and computerisation. It can be particularly helpful in investigating patients with achalasia, CREST syndrome and the other motor disorders of the oesophagus. It should not be performed in isolation but rather as an adjunct to endoscopy or radiology.

formed now, but barium swallow is an important investigation for a patient with dysphagia and may be done prior to endoscopy. It has the advantage that it can reveal pharyngeal pouches (Fig. 5), achalasia, and suggest external oesophageal compression which endoscopy does less well (Fig. 6). Endoscopy allows visualisation of oesophagitis, biopsy sampling of lesions and therapy, and will usually be required following barium swallow. If endoscopy is performed first and no cause for dysphagia is found, barium swallow should follow.

Oesophageal manometry is becoming more widely available

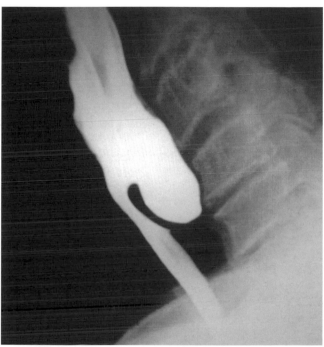

Fig. 5 **Pharyngeal pouch.**

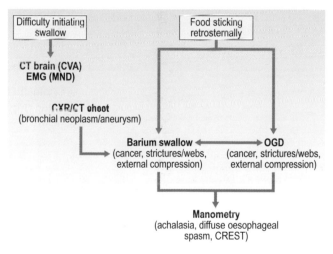

Fig. 4 **Investigative algorithm for dysphagia.**

The clinical approach

- Progressive dysphagia in the elderly is most frequently due to oesophageal cancer and investigation is mandatory.
- Neurological causes of dysphagia usually have obvious associated clinical signs at presentation.
- Upper GI endoscopy is probably the most useful first investigation although a barium swallow examination may be required also.
- Manometry can help confirm a diagnosis of achalasia and demonstrate oesophageal dysfunction in diffuse oesophageal spasm or systemic sclerosis.

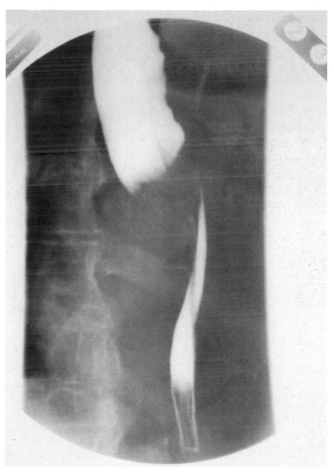

Fig. 6 **External compression of oesophagus.**

CANCER OF THE OESOPHAGUS

RELEVANT ANATOMY

The mucosa of the oesophagus is non-keratinised stratified squamous epithelium for the majority of its length and changes to gastric mucosa at the gastro-oesophageal junction. This is readily visible at endoscopy as a change from white to pink mucosa, and is approximately 40 cm from the incisor teeth (z-line or ora serrata) (Fig. 1). It follows a path in the chest behind the trachea and has the aorta wrapping round it. The close proximity to these structures means that external compression of the oesophagus can readily occur.

PATHOLOGY

Ninety-five per cent of oesophageal cancers arise from either squamous or intestinal mucosa leading to squamous cell carcinoma (SCC) or adenocarcinoma (AC) (Fig. 2). Overall, they represent 2% of all cancers and have an annual incidence of approximately 9:100 000. There has been a striking increase in the incidence of adenocarcinoma over the last 20 years, and now it represents 50% of all oesophageal carcinomas.

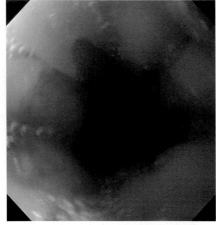

Fig. 1 **The normal gastro-oesophageal junction with change from squamous to gastric mucose at the z-line.**

SCC shows wide geographic variation in its incidence, with areas of China recording 700:100 000 annual incidence compared to 4:100 000 in the USA. This wide variation is not well understood but may relate to higher dietary intake of nitrosamines in China. Other risk factors include high alcohol consumption, particularly spirits, and tobacco usage. Achalasia, chronic peptic stricture, tylosis (rare autosomal dominant condition with hyperkeratosis of hands and soles) and Plummer–Vinson syndrome predispose to SCC.

The rise in incidence of AC may reflect an increase in Barrett's oesophagus (see pp 000–000) which carries an increased risk of up to 40% compared to the normal population. As gastric mucosa is confined normally to the distal oesophagus, it is not surprising that 80% of ACs occur in the distal oesophagus and may be difficult to distinguish from AC arising in the cardia of the stomach. AC is more frequent in men (5:1) and is less closely associated with smoking, alcohol and achalasia than SCC.

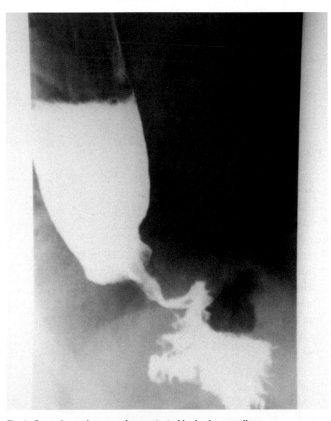

DIAGNOSIS

Oesophageal cancer is usually diagnosed late, and two thirds of patients already have meta-static disease. The decision as to whether endoscopy or barium swallow is the first investigation may depend to some extent on their availability, but if radiology suggests a tumour (Fig. 2), endoscopic biopsy will be necessary to confirm the diagnosis and aid planning of treatment.

Fig. 2 **Oesophageal cancer demonstrated by barium swallow.**

MANAGEMENT

As surgical resection is the only curative procedure for oesophageal cancer, it should at least be considered in most patients. Oesophagectomy is a major procedure and often a patient's general physical condition will preclude this. CT of the chest and abdomen is useful for detecting local invasion and metastases in the chest and liver. Endoscopic ultrasound allows assessment of depth of invasion of the oesophageal wall and local

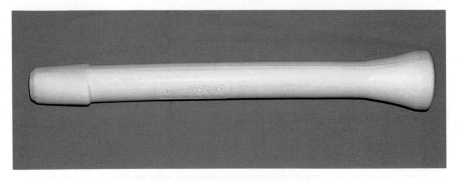

Fig. 3 **Old-fashioned rigid plastic stent for palliation of oesphageal cancer.**

node involvement, and is becoming increasingly popular for preoperative assessment.

The majority of patients, however, will not be amenable to surgery and will require palliation. The object of this is to allow patients to swallow. Malignant strictures can be dilated endoscopically with a balloon which will often produce a temporary improvement in swallowing, but dysphagia usually recurs rapidly. Endoprostheses which keep the stricture open have been around for many years. Originally, rigid plastic tubes were placed but were difficult to introduce, inflexible and often uncomfortable for the patient

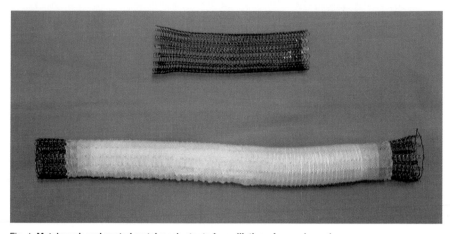

Fig. 4 **Metal mesh and coated metal mesh stents for palliation of oesophagael cancer.**

(Fig. 3). Self-expanding metal mesh stents can now be placed easily under radiological control and offer much better palliation. If a tracheo-oesophageal fistula is present, coated stents can be placed to close the fistula (Fig. 4). With a stent in place, patients will be able to tolerate fluids and small solids; large pieces of meat will usually not pass a stent and may cause bolus obstruction. Severe reflux is usual if the gastro-oesophageal junction is crossed and patients should be advised to avoid eating meals shortly before going to bed and use proton pump inhibitors. Drinking carbonated drinks during and after meals may also help ease food down. In-growth of tumour through the stent often occurs after some months and the passage can be cored out using a number of different techniques such as argon beam photocoagulation, laser light or injection of absolute alcohol. Photodynamic therapy (PDT) involves administering a photosensitising agent (such as a porphyrin) which is taken up by the tumour. The tumour is then bathed in gentlebut sustained laser which leads to tumour necrosis. This can be curative in very early mucosal lesions. Occasionally overgrowth of tumour at the proximal end of the stent can be treated by insertion of a second stent inside the first (Fig. 5). Radiotherapy may be useful in SCC for palliation. Chemotherapy is being evaluated in AC, particularly as adjuvant therapy with surgery.

Surgery of the mid-oesophagus requires thoracotomy and has an increased associated mortality – low oesophageal lesions may be approached via the abdomen and carry less operative risk.

Mean survival is 10 months, and 5-year survival is 10% which has not improved significantly recently. Attention should be paid to nutritional requirements, and liquid dietary supplementation is helpful. Salivary secretion can been reduced by the use of hyoscine, and this may make terminal patients more comfortable. Aspiration pneumonia is the most

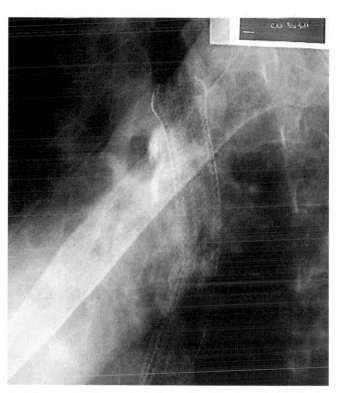

Fig. 5 **Two metal mesh stents in situ in a patient with a long oesophageal cancer.**

common cause of death, often with the patients having developed severe cachexia.

Following the initial diagnosis, if curative surgery is not possible, often a palliative stent is placed. Despite this offering comparatively good palliation, patients and families often need considerable support from the palliative care team and the gastroenterologist, who should make themselves available for further treatments such as vulgaration of tumour in-growth or nutritional advice.

Cancer of the oesophagus

- The likeliest cause of dysphagia and weight loss in an elderly person is oesophageal cancer.
- Adenocarcinoma is rising in incidence and may be due to a rise in the incidence of Barrett's oesophagus.
- Barium meal may be used first and endoscopy performed subsequently for biopsy and therapy in dysphagia.
- The majority of patients are inoperable at presentation and need palliation.
- Flexible metal stents can be placed easily and offer reasonable palliation.

DISORDERS OF THE DISTAL OESOPHAGUS

BARRETT'S OESOPHAGUS

Although not a cause of dysphagia directly, Barrett's oesophagus is included in this section because of its relationship to adenocarcinoma (AC). First described 40 years ago, there has been growing interest in this condition as its role in the development of AC is better appreciated.

PATHOLOGY

Definition of Barrett's oesophagus is evolving but the underlying change is of a metaplasia from native squamous epithelium to columnar intestinal mucosa. This may show changes associated with either gastric or small bowel mucosa, or a mixture of both. For it to be Barrett's oesophagus, there previously had to be encroachment by greater than 3 cm of columnar mucosa into the tubular oesophagus above the anatomic oesophago-gastric junction (OGJ). However, it now appears that shorter segments of Barrett's oesophagus may also predispose to AC and a better definition may be specialised columnar epithelium in the tubular oesophagus at any level.

AETIOLOGY

The aetiology of the metaplastic change is not clear but it appears to be related to reflux of gastric contents – not acid alone as acid suppression therapy does not appear to lead to a regression of the

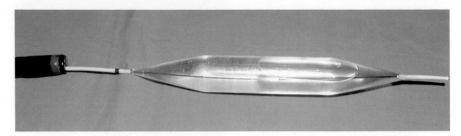

Fig. 2 **Endoscopic balloon for oesophageal dilatation passed through the endoscope and inflated.**

metaplasia, nor does anti-reflux surgery. Duodeno-oesophageal reflux has been implicated, as it contains pancreatic secretions and bile which may be pathogenic.

DIAGNOSIS

The endoscopic appearance of Barrett's mucosa varies. There may be simply a proximal migration of the z-line into the oesophagus, or the z-line may appear irregular with tongues of pink intestinal mucosa stretching into the white squamous epithelium. There may also be 'mucosal islands' of squamous epithelium in areas of pink intestinal metaplastic epithelium (Fig. 1).

PROGRESSION

Barrett's oesophagus confers an approximate increased risk of developing carcinoma of 40 times compared to the normal population, and AC has a 13% prevalence in patients with Barrett's oesophagus. There is a sequence of dysplastic changes which develop prior to AC. High-grade dysplasia detected at screening is frequently associated with AC in situ in resection specimens and may be an indication for oesophagectomy. One-third of patients with high-grade dysplasia go on to develop AC within 5 years.

MANAGEMENT

There is an intuitive attraction for screening patients with Barrett's oesophagus; however, compelling data to support its usefulness is scant. An estimated 1 case of AC is detected per 125 years of annual follow-up. Certainly there can be little merit in screening patients who would

not be fit or would decline oesophagectomy. In patients in whom screening is undertaken it is recommended that multiple biopsies are taken from each quadrant at 2 cm intervals along the length of the Barrett's epithelium in order to try and overcome the problem of patchy areas of dysplasia. Methylene blue can be used to highlight areas of dysplasia at endoscopy.

Acid suppression therapy and surgical fundoplication do not appear to reverse the dysplasia. Photodynamic therapy (PDT) is under current evaluation but appears to have the drawback that under regenerated squamous epithelium there can be areas of buried metaplastic tissue.

PEPTIC STRICTURE

Prolonged untreated acid reflux can result in the development of a peptic

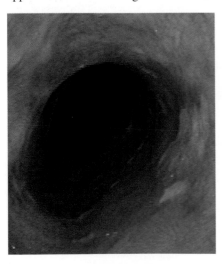

Fig. 1 **Endoscopic appearance of Barrett's oesophagus (pink areas).**

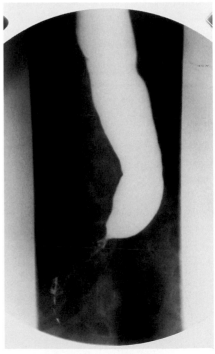

Fig. 3 **Achalasia demonstrated with a barium swallow showing dilated oesophagus above a smooth narrowing.**

stricture. Effective acid suppression therapy over the last 20 years has meant that peptic stricture is much less common. They usually occur in the distal oesophagus and can be difficult to distinguish from malignant strictures. All strictures require biopsy and benign histology does not exclude malignancy, due to sampling error. Strictures which recur quickly after dilatation are particularly suspicious of malignancy. Using pneumatic balloons that can be passed through the endoscope, dilatation can be effectively performed and, once done, stricturing is unlikely to recur with acid suppression therapy (Fig. 2).

ACHALASIA

Normally the lower oesophageal sphincter LOS relaxes ahead of a prepulsive peristaltic wave. In achalasia there is failure of the LOS to relax, accompanied by inadequate oesophageal peristalsis, causing a functional obstruction of the lower oesophagus. Consequently food and fluid accumulate in the oesophagus, which becomes progressively more dilated. Patients complain of dysphagia and 30% have respiratory problems related to aspiration of oesophageal contents.

There appears to be damage of the intramural oesophageal nerve plexus with loss of inhibitory fibres; however, the cause of this is unknown. There is an annual incidence of 1:200000, it is equally common in males and females and usually presents between the third and fifth decades.

DIAGNOSIS

Diagnosis is best made with a combination of investigations. Endoscopy may show a grossly dilated oesophagus with food debris, but there may be more subtle changes in early disease with just a mildly dilated oesophagus and an LOS which does not readily relax. This is another case where barium swallow can be helpful (Fig. 3). Oesophageal manometry has characteristic changes with aperistalsis and incomplete LOS relaxation (Fig. 4). It is important to recognise that distal oesophageal cancers can mimic achalasia either by causing external compression or by malignant cell

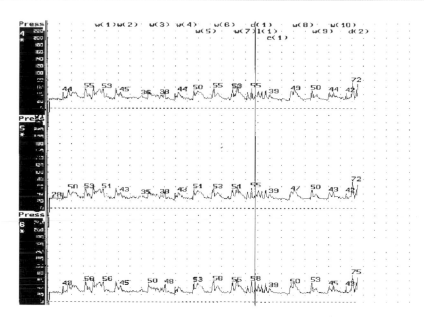

Fig. 4 **Aperistalsis demonstrated by manometry in achalasia. Note absence of significant waves.**

infiltration of the mural plexus causing similar barium and manometry changes. It is therefore essential to perform endoscopy and biopsy in suspected cases.

MANAGEMENT

The object of treatment is to facilitate swallowing, and this can be done by disrupting the circular muscle at the distal oesophagus endoscopically with pneumatic dilatation (Fig. 5). This is readily performed but carries a 5% risk of oesophageal perforation. It is effective in the majority of patients but symptoms can recur. Previously, thoracotomy was necessary to perform a surgical myotomy, but this can now be done with minimally invasive techniques and is becoming more attractive. Botulinum toxin can be injected into the distal oesophagus at endoscopy and is currently under evaluation.

Achalasia may be complicated by

the development of squamous cell carcinomas, particularly in untreated cases, but the risk is low.

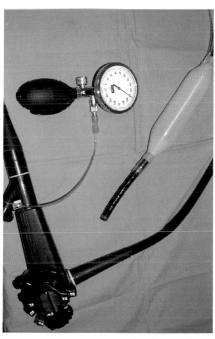

Fig. 5 **Witzel balloon on a gastroscope inflated for pneumatic dilatation of oesophagus.**

Barrett's oesophagus/peptic stricture/achalasia

- Barrett's oesophagus predisposes to AC, and its rising prevalence may account for the increased incidence of AC.
- Peptic stricture is becoming less frequent, and following dilatation recurrence can usually be prevented by effective acid suppression therapy.
- Achalasia causes a functional distal oesophageal obstruction, due to failure of the LOS to relax during swallowing. It may be missed at endoscopy, and barium swallow should be considered in patients with dysphagia and 'normal' endoscopy.
- Endoscopic biopsy is essential in Barrett's oesophagus, peptic stricture and achalasia in order to exclude malignancy.

NEUROLOGICAL AND INFECTIVE CAUSES OF DYSPHAGIA

NORMAL SWALLOWING

In normal swallowing there are two major components. The first is voluntary and involves moving the food bolus to the oropharynx. This initiates an involuntary secondary phase whereby the upper oesophageal sphincter relaxes (cricopharyngeus muscle), a prepulsive peristaltic wave forces the bolus down the length of the oesophagus and the lower oesophageal sphincter relaxes allowing the bolus into the stomach. Neurological control for the voluntary component originates in the swallowing centre located in the brain stem, with efferent impulses travelling via trigeminal, facial, hypoglossal and vagus nerves. Control of the involuntary phase is less well understood but is predominantly controlled by the intramural nerve plexus in the oesophageal wall.

CEREBROVASCULAR ACCIDENTS

Difficulty in swallowing is a common complication of cerebrovascular accidents (CVAs). It may be as a result of damage to the swallowing centre in the brain stem or motor nuclei controlling striated muscle in the hypopharynx. In some patients it is transient and frequent careful testing of swallowing is required after CVA. It is important to ensure that swallowing is safe in order to avoid aspiration and the often fatal complication of pneumonia in these debilitated patients. Many have unsatisfactory recovery of swallowing and require alternative measures for hydration and feeding. In the short term, intravenous or subcutaneous fluids are sufficient, or a nasogastric (NG) tube can be placed, but beyond approximately 2 weeks, if there is no recovery of swallowing, consideration should be given to placement of an enteral feeding tube. Percutaneous endoscopic gastrostomy (PEG) feeding tubes are popular as they have a number of advantages over NG feeding. They are readily placed, without general anaesthesia, are comfortable for patients and convenient for carers. Previous gastric surgery or ascites may preclude the placement of PEG tubes. Otherwise, fol-

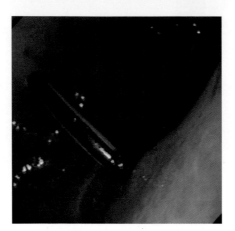

Fig. 1 **Cannula visible within stomach.**

lowing consent from the patient or relatives, the patient is sedated and gastroscoped. The optimal position for the PEG tube is decided by transillumination from the stomach and by pressure externally which is visible within the stomach. Local anaesthesia is given and a cannula placed through the abdominal wall into the stomach (Fig. 1). A guiding string is passed from the exterior to the stomach lumen and grabbed by the endoscopist who pulls it out through the mouth. The PEG tube is attached to the string and then pulled back into the stomach, through the abdominal wall. A balloon or flange prevents the PEG tube being pulled out (Fig. 2). Water can be given the day after placement and feed 24 hours after that (Fig. 3). However, it should be recognised that the 30-day mortality following PEG placement may be 10% or higher, which reflects the severity of the underlying conditions in the patients that have them placed. They last up to a year and then can be readily

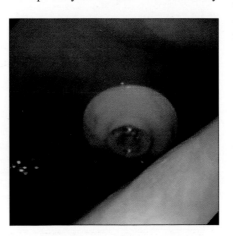

Fig. 2 **Intragastric view of PEG tube flange.**

replaced, but if sufficient recovery occurs such that they are no longer required they can be removed endoscopically.

The selection of patients who are suitable for PEG placement represents a clinical challenge. If a patient has had a dense CVA and prognosis is very poor then it may be inappropriate to offer PEG placement. Other neurological conditions that may result in difficulty in swallowing, such as Parkinson's disease, may also be suitable for PEG placement. Difficulty arises when demented patients are not eating and drinking sufficiently. A PEG tube would help this but not the underlying condition. The procedure-related mortality is particularly high and most clinicians agree that PEG placement in this situation would be inappropriate.

PARKINSON'S DISEASE

Degeneration in the swallowing centre in Parkinson's disease often leads to failure of upper oesophageal sphincter relaxation. This is usually successfully treated by conventional anti-Parkinson's medication.

MISCELLANEOUS NEUROLOGICAL CONDITIONS

Multiple sclerosis and motor neurone disease may result in brain stem damage and swallowing difficulty. In such patients PEG tube feeding is an option.

Neuromuscular diseases such as myasthenia gravis and polymyositis may cause dysphagia via the effects on striated muscle and will often respond to medical therapy.

INFECTIONS OF THE OESOPHAGUS

Candida albicans

Candida albicans is a commensal which only becomes invasive when there is impairment of the host defence mechanism. In the oesophagus these mechanisms normally comprise saliva, oesophageal motility, refluxing acid, and healthy epithelium. They may be disturbed by antibiotics, impaired immunity (such as in medication for transplantation), AIDS, chemotherapy, and in diabetes mellitus, alcoholism, steroid and acid suppression therapy, and with age.

Invasive *Candida* causes an oesophagitis which usually results in painful swallowing and retrosternal pain. There is frequently evidence of oral *Candida*.

Diagnosis is usually made at endoscopy when there are adherent white plaques with an advancing margin, which when removed show a raw mucosa (Fig. 4). Confirmation is with brush cytology. Treatment can be with topically active agents such as nystatin, absorbed agents such as fluconazole or, in the severely ill, intravenous amphotericin B.

Herpes simplex virus (HSV)

HSV infection is usually seen in the immunocompromised patient. It results in pain on swallowing and retrosternal pain. Infection results in small shallow ulcers with a raised margin and is diagnosed by tissue culture from biopsies taken from the edge of the ulcer. Treatment is with anti-viral agents such as acyclovir.

Cytomegalovirus (CMV)

CMV oesophagitis is similar to HSV in that it usually occurs in the immunocompromised patient and results in oesophageal ulceration in the distal oesophagus. Ulcers are large and shallow. Tissue culture confirms the diagnosis and treatment is with ganciclovir.

CORROSIVE DAMAGE OF THE OESOPHAGUS

This follows ingestion of caustic agents either deliberately or accidentally, and causes most damage proximally in the oesophagus. Gastric lavage should usually be avoided to prevent secondary oesophageal damage. Acid suppression may be useful following the trauma but complications such as strictures may occur.

Pills may lodge in the oesophagus and cause discrete ulceration, particularly if the patient takes them immediately prior to lying down or if there is abnormal oesophageal motility. Potassium pills and antibiotics are the most frequent offenders.

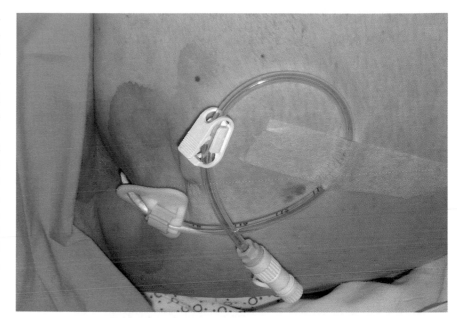

Fig. 3 **External view of PEG tube.**

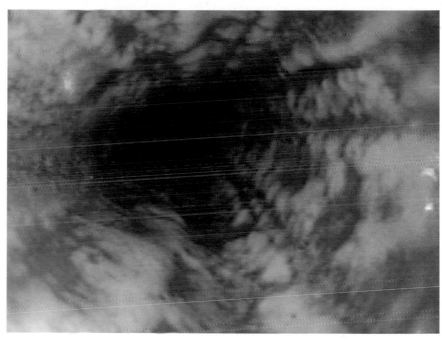

Fig. 4 **Oesophageal *Candida*.**

Neurological and infective causes of dysphagia

- Swallowing has an initial voluntary component which places the food bolus in the oropharynx and is followed by an involuntary upper oesophageal sphincter relaxation, a prepulsive peristaltic wave through the length of the oesophagus and then lower oesophageal sphincter relaxation.
- CVAs are the most common neurological cause of dysphagia.
- PEG placement facilitates enteral feeding in patients in need of long-term feeding.
- *Candida* is usually readily recognised at endoscopy by discrete white plaques, and may reflect impaired immunity in the patient.
- HSV and CMV infections usually occur in the immunocompromised patient and cause painful dysphagia. Discrete shallow ulceration is typical.
- Pills may lodge in the oesophagus and cause ulceration, resulting in painful dysphagia.

THE CLINICAL APPROACH

HISTORY

Heartburn

Eliciting a history relating to the oesophagus from a patient is usually straightforward. Heartburn is the most common symptom and is described as a retrosternal burning pain which may radiate up into the throat or down into the epigastrium. It has probably been experienced by all adults and occurs monthly in up to one-third of the population. Twenty-five per cent of pregnant women experience heartburn daily.

Heartburn is frequently worsened when the intra-abdominal pressure is raised by straining, bending or stooping. It is worse after heavy meals and certain dietary elements such as fatty foods and chocolate may worsen the symptoms by lowering the lower oesophageal sphincter (LOS) pressure. Citrus fruit and spicy foods may aggravate symptoms by causing direct mucosal irritation. Tobacco smoking seems to worsen symptoms by increasing oesophageal acid clearance time and by decreasing production of alkaline saliva which has a neutralising effect. Drugs such as beta-blockers, theophyllines, calcium channel blockers and drugs with anticholinergic side-effects all may worsen heartburn by reducing the LOS pressure or decreasing oesophageal peristalsis. Anxiety may worsen symptoms by creating increased patient awareness and sensitivity.

Heartburn is caused by reflux of gastric contents which are acidic and contain injurious agents such as pepsin and bile salts. Heartburn symptoms do not correspond well with the severity of acid reflux when measured with pH monitoring nor do symptoms correlate well with the degree of mucosal damage. Heartburn is a symptom and should not be confused with oesophagitis although both may co-exist.

Odynophagia

Pain associated with swallowing is a much less common symptom. Hot and spicy foods may cause direct irritation and the symptom usually reflects severe oesophageal inflammation or ulceration. This may be caused by pill-induced oesophagitis, infectious oesophagitis (*Candida*, herpes or CMV) or peptic ulceration.

Belching

This procedure expels gas ingested whilst eating and does not usually present a problem. However, in a number of patients there is incessant noisy regurgitation of air which occurs throughout the day. It frequently becomes highly distressing both to patients and their families and can be difficult to manage. Contrary to popular belief, it is not particularly associated with hiatus hernia or gall-bladder disease. It represents abnormal air swallowing (aerophagia) and is usually a functional disorder when not associated with more sinister symptoms.

Non-cardiac chest pain

Occasionally it is impossible to distinguish between oesophageal and cardiac chest pain (Fig. 1). There are shared neural pathways via the vagus nerve and oesophageal pain may be described as tight or crushing in nature. However, pointers towards an oesophageal cause include nocturnal symptoms wakening patients from sleep, a relationship to swallowing, particularly hot or cold foodstuffs, and no exacerbation by exercise.

It is not absolutely clear how this symptom is produced but it may reflect oesophageal spasm. Cardiac pain should be recognisable by its character and relationship to exercise. Musculoskeletal pain is usually a sharp pain, localised to one spot, worsened by

Table 1 **LA classification for reflux oesophagitis**

Grade A	One (or more) mucosal break no longer than 5 mm that does not extend between the tops of two mucosal folds
Grade B	One (or more) mucosal break more than 5 mm long, that does not extend between the tops of two mucosal folds
Grade C	One (or more) mucosal break that is continuous between the tops of two or more mucosal folds, but which involves less than 75% of the cicumference
Grade A	One (or more) mucosal break, which involves at least 75% of the oesophageal cicumference

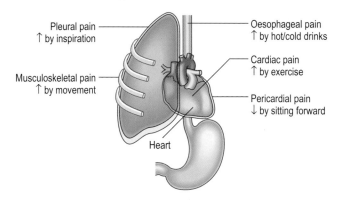

Fig. 1 **Sources of chest pain and clues to their source in history.**

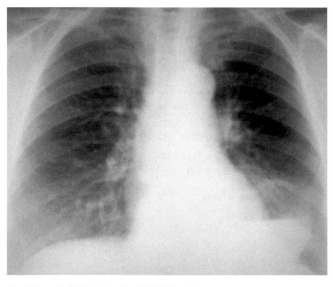

Fig. 2 **Impacted hiatus hernia with fluid level.**

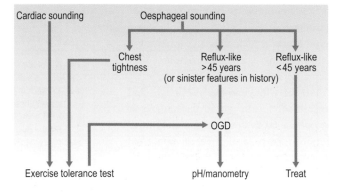

Fig. 3 **Investigative alogrithm – chest pain.**

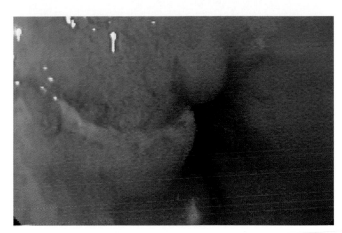

Fig. 4 **Reflux oesophagitis.**

movement or adopting certain positions, and tenderness to touch. Pleuritic pain is described as sharp and worsened by deep inspiration, and there may be an associated pleural rub. If no convincing distinction can be made between a cardiac or oesophageal cause for the pain, it is reasonable to try to exclude a cardiac cause first as this has the most serious implications for the patient if missed.

EXAMINATION

This is usually unrewarding but in the presence of severe acid reflux back into the mouth, there may be damaged dentition. Obesity is common and correlates with reflux symptoms. Rarely, bowel sounds can be heard within the chest when there is a large diaphragmatic hiatus with bowel herniated into the chest cavity (Fig. 2). A cardiac cause for the chest pain may be more likely if there is evidence of peripheral vascular disease or cardiac disease such as aortic stenosis. If aortic stenosis is suspected, echocardiography should be performed first as an exercise test carries the serious risk of sudden death.

INVESTIGATION (Fig. 3)

In many patients, it may be inappropriate to investigate symptoms of reflux, particularly in pregnant women or in the young, and symptomatic treatment is all that is necessary.

Upper GI endo-scopy is the most valuable first inve-stigation. It can confirm the presence of oeso-phagitis or other consequences of gastro-oesophageal reflux such as Barrett's oesophagus and stricture formation (Fig. 4). Ulceration as a result of infection, medication or inges-tion of caustics can also be demonstrated. Patients are occasionally disappointed if no oesophagitis is shown and it should be explained to them that this does not belittle their symptoms.

Many endoscopic grading systems are in use and Table 1 outlines a common one, which may be useful in research projects, but a simpler description is more effective in the clinical setting.

Acid reflux can be quantified using pH monitoring (Table 2 and Fig. 5). pH probes are placed proximal to the LOS and allowed to monitor pH for prolonged periods — usually 24 hours. pH of less than 4 is considered abnormal and a total time of greater than 4.2% is prolonged. This also allows timing of maximal reflux whether it be post prandial, nocturnal or daytime and allows the investigator to determine whether reflux episodes correspond with symptoms.

Oesophageal manometry is normally performed prior to pH monitoring and allows identification and positioning of the LOS, and assessment of oesophageal peristalsis and LOS relaxation.

Manometry and pH monitoring are not usually necessary but are helpful in diagnosis where the history and investigations are unclear and as a prelude to surgical intervention for gastro-oesophageal reflux disease (GORD).

Infusion of acid into the distal oesophagus can be performed in order to reproduce chest pain (Bernstein test) although the diagnostic usefulness of this test is questionable.

Occasionally it is necessary to investigate a cardiac cause for a patient's symptoms, even if an oesophageal cause is suggested by the history. Exercise tolerance testing is the most useful first investigation, but its limitations, particularly in the younger age group and in women, should be remembered.

Table 2 **PH study: normal values pH studies**

Normal value	
Percent time below pH 4.0	4.2%
Duration of longest episode	9.2 minutes
Number of episodes	<50
Number of episodes longer than 5 minutes	≤3

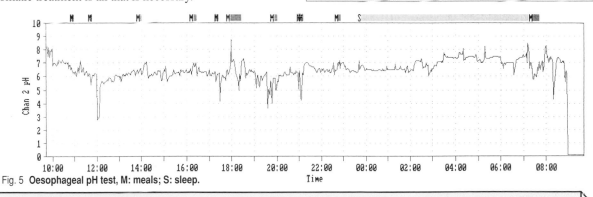

Fig. 5 **Oesophageal pH test, M: meals; S: sleep.**

The clinical approach

- Heartburn is the commonest symptom attributable to the oesophagus and is easily recognized by its nature.
- Simple GORD in the young without accompanying sinister features may be treated symptomatically without investigation.

- Oesophageal spasm may be difficult to distinguish from cardiac pain and require more invasive investigation; however, it is usually prudent to try to exclude cardiac pain first.

- GORD and heart disease are both common and may co-exist in the same patient.
- Repeated, troublesome belching is not usually associated with GI pathology and is most frequently 'functional'.

GASTRO-OESOPHAGEAL REFLUX DISEASE

Gastro-oesophageal reflux disease (GORD) is a term used to include patients who suffer with symptoms of reflux, with or without oesophagitis or any other complication of acid reflux, and who mayor may not have a hiatus hernia. Oesophagitis ranges from minor microscopic changes of an acute inflammatory infiltrate with neutrophils and eosinophils to mucosal erosions and ulceration. As the damaging agents are luminal, damage is predominantly mucosal and perforation is unusual.

Normally, prevention of acid damage is achieved by a combination of physiological barriers. The LOS is a 3–4 cm long collection of smooth muscle fibres which maintains a resting tone of 10–30 mmHg pressure. There is also extrinsic pressure exerted from the crura of the diaphragm at the same point and the angle of His (the angle of entry of the oesophagus into the stomach) which both help retain acid within the stomach. Periods of LOS relaxation occur in all individuals and allow transient reflux of acid into the oesophagus. This initiates a distal oesophageal peristaltic wave which progressively clears the acid. Swallowed saliva is alkaline and also helps neutralise oesophageal acid (Fig. 1).

It is probably true that there is no single failure of any one of these preventative mechanisms in GORD and the disease probably reflects a combination of them. Hiatus hernia (displacement of the LOS into the chest) is extremely common and many patients attribute GORD to its presence, but it is probably only a minor contributory factor.

Symptomatic reflux is usually accompanied by no oesophageal mucosal changes and the severity of symptoms does not correlate with the presence or abscence of oeso-phagitis; however, duration of acid exposure is related to the degree of oesophagitis. Chronic reflux may result in stricture formation and the development of Barrett's oesophagus. Recent work has suggested that long-term, severe reflux significantly increases the chance of developing oesophageal adenocarcinoma.

Acid reflux may be associated with extra-oesophageal manifestations and has been associated with asthma, chronic cough, hoarseness and nocturnal choking. Dentists may see severe enamel damage as a result of chronic acid reflux.

MANAGEMENT

GORD is a chronic relapsing condition with more than 80% of patients having a recurrence within 6 months of discontinuation of medication. The majority of sufferers do not seek medical attention and tend to self-medicate with over the counter antacids, alginates and H_2 receptor antagonists (H_2RAs).

When medical help is sought lifestyle changes should be advised and can result in symptomatic improvement. These include weight reduction, stopping smoking, avoidance of large meals and excessive alcohol and elevation of the head end of the bed by 20 cm, particularly for nocturnal symptoms. However, these measures are more difficult to achieve and patients frequently prefer to use medication rather than lose weight or stop smoking. Alginates (e.g. Gaviscon or Gastrocote) have the advantage over antacids in that they both have a neutralising

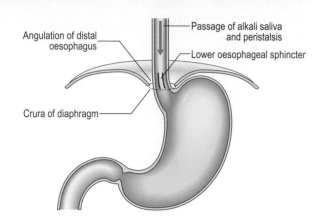

Fig. 1 **Mechanism of protection of oesophagus from acid reflux.**

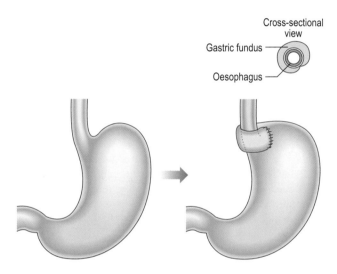

Fig. 2 **Nissen fundoplication.**

effect and also form a protective raft above the gastric contents which creates a physical barrier between acid and mucosa. H_2RAs (e.g. ranitidine or cimetidine) are an effective treatment and doses should be titrated against symptoms. Promotility agents (e.g. metoclopramide) act by increasing gastric peristalsis and increasing LOS tone. They have moderate efficacy and may be used in conjunction with acid suppression therapy in resistant cases. The advent of proton pump inhibitors (PPIs) (e.g. omeprazole or lansoprazole) have re-duced the importance of H_2RAs in the treatment of severe disease as PPIs are undoubtedly superior in acid suppression and therefore efficacy in GORD. As a result of the relapsing nature of the condition and the efficacy of PPIs, patients are often reluctant to discontinue medication. This produces concerns about long-term drug usage and also has health and economic implications.

In part because of this and as a result of improvement in surgical techniques, surgical treatment of patients with GORD is increasing. Fundoplication (Fig. 2) was previously a major thoracic and abdominal procedure. Laparoscopic techniques allow the same operation to be performed with the advantage of it being less invasive. Fundoplication is effective in treating reflux symptoms and some of their consequences such as oesophagitis, but not Barrett's oesophagus. It carries a recognized morbidity, particularly dysphagia, and should be considered only in young patients in whom medical treatment has failed or who require continuous acid suppression therapy.

OESOPHAGEAL CAUSES OF CHEST PAIN

After GORD, oesophageal dysmotility comprises the largest group of causes of non-cardiac chest pain, and may be diagnosed in 25% of patients with non-cardiac chest pain. Several motor abnormalities of the oesophagus are now recognised because of their specific manometric characteristics. The mechanisms by which these conditions cause chest pain are not clear, but seem to involve pain generated by oesophageal distension, a reduced sensory threshold to oesophageal distension in some patients, or, less likely, impaired blood flow during high amplitude contractions.

Nutcracker oesophagus

This is recognised by the finding of mean distal oesophageal pressures during wet swallows of greater than 180 mmHg. These high pressures which exceed systemic blood pressure were thought to impair oesophageal blood flow and hence cause pain, but the complex blood supply and brief duration of these peaks suggest that this is not the cause (Fig. 3).

Non-specific oesophageal dysmotility

Weak or poorly conducted peristaltic waves characterise this disorder and sufferers may also experience oesophageal chest pain. It is important to recognise this abnormality prior to anti-reflux surgery as poor peristalsis increases the likelihood of postoperative dysphagia.

Diffuse oesophageal spasm

Following dry swallows, peristaltic waves are frequently non-progressive but when water is swallowed, less than 20% should be non-peristaltic or simultaneous. If the percentage is greater than this, the motility changes of diffuse oesophageal spasm are confirmed. There may be other associated abnormalities such as multi-peaked or prolonged contractions.

TREATMENT

As GORD represents the major cause of non-cardiac chest pain, it is reasonable to consider a trial of acid suppression therapy in patients in whom a cardiac cause seems unlikely. If this fails, patients may respond to nitrates or calcium channel blockers for their pain, although they can be a difficult group to treat.

RUPTURED OESOPHAGUS

The commonest cause of oesophageal perforation was previously forceful vomiting often with attempted suppression of the act (Boerhaave's syndrome), resulting in distal oesophageal perforation. Perforation following instrumentation of the oesophagus now accounts for over 50% of cases of oesophageal rupture following either endoscopy or, more frequently, dilatation for strictures.

Symptoms are of pain within either the chest, or the neck for more proximal perforations, and there may be odynophagia. Signs include subcutaneous crepitation (surgical emphysema), pleural effusion, or a crunching noise associated with heart sounds. Chest X-ray may show mediastinal gas or widening, pleural effusion or subcutaneous gas. Contrast radiology should be performed, usually using a water-soluble contrast medium first. This has the advantage that if it leaks into the chest cavity, it is more readily absorbed than barium but the disadvantage that if aspirated, it invokes a severe pulmonary reaction.

MANAGEMENT

Small leaks that are discovered early and where there has been spontaneous resealing may be treated non-operatively with intravenous antibiotics, fluid, and maintaining the patient nil by mouth. Larger leaks or where abscesses have formed require surgical intervention with drainage, repair of the tear or even resection. When perforation has complicated dilatation for oesophageal cancer, the lesion may be sealed with a plastic-coated, expandable metal stent placed endoscopically. Despite these measures, oesophageal leaks carry a high mortality and should be diagnosed as soon as possible and considered following any complicated oesophageal procedure.

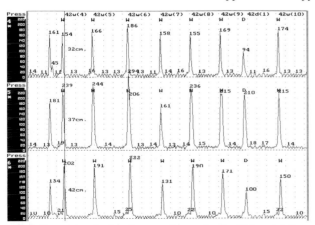

Fig. 3 **Manometry of nutcracker oesophagus showing high peristaltic pressures.**

Gastro-oesophageal reflux disease
- Symptoms of GORD do not correlate with endoscopic findings of oesophagitis, but oesophagitis does reflect the degree of acid reflux.
- Hoarse voice, cough, nocturnal choking and asthma may accompany severe reflux.
- Lifestyle advice may be helpful but GORD is a relapsing condition that often requires long-term treatment.
- Laparoscopic fundoplication may be useful in long-term management of patients with intractable GORD.
- Oesophageal chest pain can be difficult to diagnose but is found in a significant proportion of patients with a non-cardiac cause for their pain.
- Ruptured oesophagus must always be considered when patients develop chest pain after vomiting.

THE CLINICAL APPROACH

An acute abdomen is recognised by its sudden onset, localisation of pain within the abdomen and clinical findings of abdominal rigidity, guarding and absent bowel sounds. Intestinal obstruction is identified by colicky pain, abdominal distension with vomiting and absolute constipation with the finding of gaseous distension and tinkling bowel sounds on examination. Chronic recurrent abdominal pain often comes with many features which are less specific and which require the taking of a careful history to avoid unnecessary investigation and waste of time (Table 1).

HISTORY

As with any pain, the usual nine features must be elicited (Table 2). A junior doctor will probably elicit these features rote fashion, whilst the more experienced clinician will recognise patterns of pain that point to certain diagnoses (Table 3).

With pains that have been troubling the patient for several weeks it is necessary to establish whether they are continuous – occurring both day and night, and whether they have been worsening, have remained unchanged or are improving. Relentless pains may indicate a malignant process which tends not to have periods of improvement, but gradually worsens. Episodic pain that has periods of painlessness between attacks is suggestive of biliary or gallbladder disease (Fig. 1), peptic disorders (Fig. 2), benign pancreatic disorders and functional bowel syndromes.

Weight loss is a good predictor of organic disease and occurs with neoplastic conditions, in conditions where pain is aggravated by food and in chronic inflammatory conditions. Changes in bowel habit or rectal bleeding suggest a colonic cause for the pain. Rigors are associated with infections in the biliary and renal tracts.

Having established the features of the pain, it is still essential to obtain a full history, including information regarding past medical history, alcohol and drugs, and it can offer an insight into a patient's anxieties if enquiry is made into what the patient thinks is the cause of the pain. This may also be helpful in later manage-

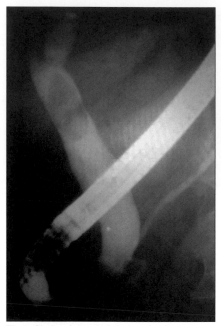

Fig. 1 **Cholangiogram of stones showing gallstones in the CBD.**

ment if it is possible to specifically allay a fear, particularly that of cancer.

It is not unusual for the first set of investigations to fail to yield a diagnosis; indeed, in some conditions such as irritable bowel syndrome there are no confirmatory investigations available. It always serves the clinician well to retake the essential components of the history, as on retelling, the patient's description may change, suggesting an alternative diagnosis to the one originally considered and thus leading in a different direction of investigation. Alternatively, re-establishing the history may confirm the clinician's previously held view.

EXAMINATION

If examination is limited to the abdomen alone, systemic signs will be missed and a more general examination is always recommended. Site of pain can be identified as can areas of tenderness (Fig. 3). Masses when felt should be characterised in the traditional manner (Table 4).

Often the clinical examination will yield no clinical signs, which only serves to stress the importance of the history, as the investigation plan will often be formed without positive clinical signs.

INVESTIGATIONS (Fig. 4)

It is usual to perform a sequence of blood tests including a full blood count (FBC),

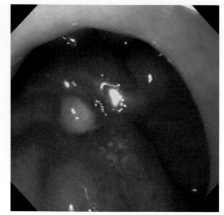

Fig. 2 **Peptic ulcer.**

biochemistry and liver function tests. A raised serum calcium level can lead to abdominal pain; diabetes can present with abdominal pain, but patients are usually acutely unwell when they present in this form. Inflammatory markers such as erythrocyte sedimentation rate (ESR) and C-reactive protein (CRP) may be helpful. Measurement of urinary porphyrins is required for acute porphyrias.

Table 1 **Clinical features of the acute abdomen and intestinal obstruction**

Acute abdomen
Severe, localised constant pain
Sudden onset
Abdominal rigidity and guarding
Absent bowel sounds
Intestinal abdomen
Colicky pain
Gradual onset
Vomiting/absolute constipation
Abdominal distension
Tinkling bowel sounds

Table 2 **Features to be documented of an abdominal pain**

1	**Site** Identify area of abdomen (and depth of pain)
2	**Onset** Sudden, gradual, time of day
3	**Severity** Patient's assessment including effects (go to bed, not go to work, go to hospital)
4	**Nature** Burning, throbbing, stabbing, colicky, constricting, or distension
5	**Progression** May get worse, improve, stay constant or fluctuate. Is it recurrent or a single episode?
6	**Duration and ending** Length of time the pain lasted, how it disappeared (suddenly as if something had passed, gradually, following vomiting or defaecation, only with medication)
7	**Aggravating factors** Eating, posture/movement, drugs
8	**Relieving factors** Eating, posture/movement, drugs
9	**Radiation** From the original site to another such as the back

The common types of pain include dyspepsia, which will prompt upper GI investigations with gastroscopy, biliary type pain, which is best investigated first with an ultrasound scan, and pain requiring lower GI investigations such as flexible sigmoidoscopy, barium enema or colonoscopy for pain referable to the colon. The pancreas and lesions in the transverse colon can lead to epigastric pain, which can be misinterpreted as arising from the stomach and duodenum and should be considered when gastroscopy is negative.

CT scanning, white cell scanning, and angiography can be later investigations in more obscure cases. Small bowel barium studies are required to diagnose small bowel diseases such as Crohn's disease. HIDA scanning is most useful for detecting acute cholecystitis, or biliary dysfunction in sphincter of Oddi dysfunction. Pain following cholecystectomy is quite a common clinical problem and is described as a pain in the right upper quadrant that may have an association with meals, particularly fatty foods, which radiates through to the right subscapular region. The causes include retained common bile duct stones and sphincter of Oddi dysfunction. Investigation includes ultrasound scanning, HIDA scanning and endoscopic retrograde cholangiopancreatography (ERCP).

Table 3 Clinical features of common causes of abdominal pain

	Peptic disease	Gallstone disease	Irritable bowel	Chronic pancreatitis	Pancreatic cancer
Site	Epigastric	Right upper quadrant	Generalised, may migrate	Epigastric	Epigastric
Onset	Gradual	Gradual/rapid	Gradual	Gradual	Gradual
Severity	Moderate	Moderate – severe	Mild – severe	Mild – moderate	Mild – moderate
Nature	Burning, gnawing	Colicky	Colicky	Aching	Gnawing
Progression	Variable	Variable	Variable	Variable	Relentless
Duration	Hours	Hours	Hours/days	Days	Continuous
Aggravating factors	NSAIDs, hunger	Fatty foods	Many and variable	Food, alcohol	Nil
Relieving factors	Food, antacids	Nil	Defaecation	Nil	Nil
Radiation	To back (for posterior duodenal ulcers)	To right subscapular area		To back	To back
Associated features	Nausea, pain often cyclical	Nausea, rigors with, cholangitis	Reflux, change in bowel habit	Diarrhoea, association with alcohol	Weight loss, obstructive jaundice

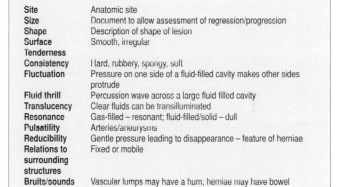

Table 4 Characteristics of a mass

Site	Anatomic site
Size	Document to allow assessment of regression/progression
Shape	Description of shape of lesion
Surface	Smooth, irregular
Tenderness	
Consistency	Hard, rubbery, spongy, soft
Fluctuation	Pressure on one side of a fluid-filled cavity makes other sides protrude
Fluid thrill	Percussion wave across a large fluid filled cavity
Translucency	Clear fluids can be transilluminated
Resonance	Gas-filled – resonant; fluid-filled/solid – dull
Pulsatility	Arteries/aneurysms
Reducibility	Gentle pressure leading to disappearance – feature of herniae
Relations to surrounding structures	Fixed or mobile
Bruits/sounds	Vascular lumps may have a hum; herniae may have bowel sounds

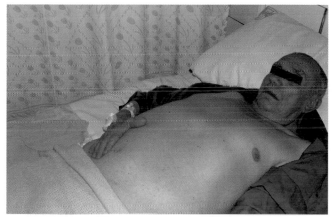

Fig. 3 **Abdominal tenderness.**

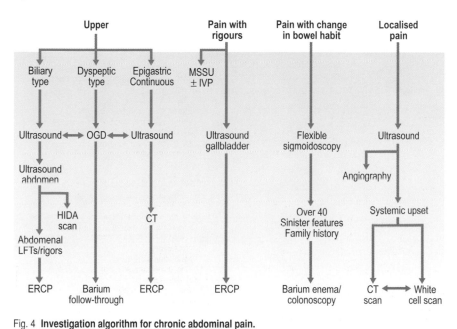

Fig. 4 **Investigation algorithm for chronic abdominal pain.**

The clinical approach

- All pains should be properly characterised.
- Careful attention to associated symptoms such as weight loss, change in bowel habit or bleeding will help direct investigation.
- Weight loss is a predictor for organic disease.
- Retaking a history may suggest an alternative route of investigation.

DYSPEPSIA

NON-ULCER DYSPEPSIA

It is not unusual for there to be confusion when a diagnosis is based on symptoms alone. This is undoubtedly the case with non-ulcer dyspepsia (NUD), but it is an essential diagnostic group because it represents up to 40% of patients who present with 'persistent or recurrent pain or discomfort that is centred in the upper abdomen or epigastrium' (dyspepsia), and in whom upper GI endoscopy and radiology are normal. Symptoms can be subdivided into:

- *Ulcer-like* dyspepsia
  Epigastric pain relieved by food, often occurring at night
- *Dysmotility-like* dyspepsia
  Upper abdominal discomfort, worse after meals, accompanied with bloating, early satiety and nausea
- *Reflux-like* dyspepsia
  Upper abdominal pain with associated reflux symptoms.

This classification has not proved helpful in tailoring therapy, except for reflux-like symptoms which might be better treated as for GORD. The pathology responsible for causing the symptoms of NUD has focused on two main areas:

1. gastric dysmotility
2. *Helicobacter pylori*-related gastritis.

During fasting, the stomach exhibits migrating motor complexes (MMCs) along with the rest of the GI tract and post-prandially shows relaxation of the gastric fundus to accommodate the food bolus. The antrum has high amplitude contractions to reduce particle size and the pylorus has phasic contractions to allow slow emptying of the stomach. There may be decreased compliance of the gastric fundus in NUD patients but this does not correlate well with symptoms, particularly nausea and early satiety, nor does it predict a good outcome with treatment using promotility agents.

H. pylori-related gastritis has come under close scrutiny in patients with NUD. There appears to be no benefit accrued by eradicating *H. pylori* in patients with NUD. Gastric acid hypersecretion does not cause NUD as basal and peak acid output is similar in both patients and controls.

MANAGEMENT

After the diagnosis of NUD, subsequent further investigation should be avoided as it implies diagnostic uncertainty and may worsen therapeutic outcome. Minimum treatment required should be adopted with simple antacids. More intractable cases may be treated with H_2 receptor antagonists or PPIs for 4–6 weeks and then discontinued and reserved for symptom recurrence. Promotility agents may be beneficial and are best taken shortly before meals. Evidence supporting the usefulness of *H. pylori* eradication in NUD patients is lacking but as peptic ulcer disease is periodic, it is possible that patients were in remission at the time of endoscopy. Consequently, it may be appropriate to offer *H. pylori* eradication therapy in patients showing relevant symptoms.

GASTRITIS

Gastritis is an endoscopic or histological diagnosis which may or may not have associated symptoms. If present, symptoms may be similar to those found in NUD but GI haemorrhage may also occur with erosive gastritis. Since the discovery of *H. pylori,* attempts have been made to establish types of gastritis.

TREATMENT

Haemorrhagic gastritis may on occasion be so severe as to warrant gastrectomy, but usually settles spontaneously. Causative agents such as drugs should be discontinued and PPIs instituted. The role of *H. pylori* eradication is necessary. Gastric atrophy is common in the elderly and treatment is only necessary with vitamin B_{12} when pernicious anaemia develops. Reflux gastritis is relatively common and may respond to promotility agents or chelators like sucralfate.

HELICOBACTER PYLORI

MICROBIOLOGY

The discovery of *H. pylori* in 1982 revolutionised the way we think of many upper GI conditions. It is a spiral, Gram-negative bacterium which has characteristic unipolar flagella and produces copious amounts of the enzyme urease. It resides predominantly in the mucous layer overlying gastric mucosa, whether this be in

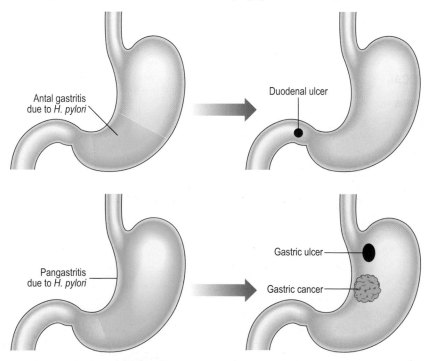

Fig. 1 **Proposed mechanism by which *H. pylori* can result in gastric ulcer/cancer or duodenal ulcer.**

layer overlying gastric mucosa, whether this be in the stomach, or in areas of gastric metaplasia in the duodenum. It survives in this hostile environment by closely adhering to the gastric epithelium and by creating a less acidic micro-environment by splitting urea to ammonia and bicarbonate. The abundance of urease is the basis of many of the methods used for detection.

EPIDEMIOLOGY

The prevalence of *H. pylori* infection in Western society is falling. Most infection is acquired in childhood after the age of 2, probably transmitted by the oral–oral or faecal–oral route and has reached a prevalence of approximately 20% by the age of 25, subsequently rising by 1% a year. In less developed countries prevalence may be 80% by the age of 20. This may reflect quality of sanitation which would account for the falling prevalence in the West. Once eradicated, re-infection is unusual and occurs at 1% per annum.

DETECTION

Invasive techniques for detecting *H. pylori* require endoscopic biopsy of gastric mucosa and allow detection by urease, culture or histology. Non-invasive techniques detect serum antibodies or exhaled radio-labelled carbon split from urea by *H. pylori* urease, and probably represent the best technique for detecting *H. pylori* when sensitivity, specificity and cost are considered (Table 1).

CLINICAL ASSOCIATIONS

Gastritis

Acute infection with *H. pylori* results in symptoms of epigastric pain and nausea associated with acute gastritis and transient hypochlorhydria. The majority of acutely infected individuals go on to develop chronic gastritis. This may ultimately affect the antrum of the stomach which is most closely associated with the development of duodenal ulceration. Alternatively, a pangastritis can occur which is associated with the development of gastric atrophy, gastric ulcer and gastric cancer. The mechanisms which determine how chronic infection develops are not clear. Chronic gastritis may be asymptomatic or have the features of NUD (Fig. 1).

Duodenal ulcer

There is evidence of a high association between *H. pylori* infection and duodenal ulcers – 95% of duodenal ulcer patients are infected with *H. pylori* and the finding that effective eradication results in the duodenal ulcer relapse rate falling from 75% to less than 5% per annum.

Gastric ulcer

When NSAIDs are excluded, up to 80% of gastric ulcers are associated with *H. pylori* and show similar falls in relapse rate following eradication therapy to those for duodenal ulcers.

Gastric cancer

In up to half of patients with chronic gastritis, atrophic gastritis and intestinal metaplasia develop. These are important precursors of gastric adenocarcinomas and are associated with *H. pylori* as it is the major cause of chronic gastritis. Chronic infection seems to increase the risk of developing gastric cancer by three- to four-fold, which is increased to an almost six-fold increased risk if Cag A antibodies (highly antigenic proteins produced by approximately 60% of *H. pylori*) are present.

Mucosa associated lymphoid tissue (MALT lymphoma)

This lymphoma, predominantly derived from B cells, is a rare gastric tumour associated with *H. pylori* and in its early stages may be cured by eradication therapy.

TREATMENT

Currently, triple therapy with a PPI and two antibiotics (e.g. amoxycillin and clarithromycin or metronidazole) is commonly used and has eradication rates up to 90%.

Confirmation of eradication is best performed by the use of a breath test, but should not be performed too early following treatment as false negative results may occur as a result of suppression rather than eradication of *H. pylori*. Antibodies to *H. pylori* take 6 months to begin to disappear which precludes serum testing to confirm eradication. Treatment failure may be due to patient non-compliance, metronidazole resistance (prevalent in women taking metronidazole as single therapy for PID) and in more urban areas. There may also be a degree of antibiotic resistance in smokers.

Table 1 **Diagnostic tests for *H. pylori* and their estimated costs.**

	Sensitivity (%)	Specificity (%)	Relative cost
Non-invasive			
Serology	88–99	86–95	£
Urea breath test	90–97	90–100	££
Invasive (requiring endoscopy)			
Rapid urease test (CLO test)	89–98	93–98	££££*
Histology	93–99	95–99	£££££*
Culture	77–92	100	£££££*
* Includes cost of endoscopy			
Taken from Secrets in GI/liver disease.			

Dyspepsia

- Non-ulcer dyspepsia is a diagnostic term that may encompass a number of conditions including gastritis and gastric dysmotility. Peptic ulceration may be the real cause of symptoms if endoscopy has been performed at a time when the ulcer has healed.
- Gastritis is a histological or endoscopic description which may or may not be associated with dyspeptic symptoms. There are many causes including drugs, alcohol and *H. pylori* and all should be considered.
- *H. pylori* is an infection usually acquired in childhood and which persists through life.
- *H. pylori* is closely associated with gastritis, and duodenal and gastric ulceration and may be important in the development of gastric cancer.
- Eradication of *H. pylori* results in ulcer healing and vastly lower recurrence rate compared to ulcers healed simply with acid suppression therapy.

PEPTIC ULCER DISEASE

NORMAL GASTRIC SECRETION AND DEFENCE

The gastric mucosa is separated into different functional areas. Glands within the cardia produce predominantly mucus. In the fundus and body, the parietal (oxyntic) glands contain parietal cells which produce hydrogen ions and intrinsic factor; chief cells which produce pepsinogen; and endocrine (ECL) cells, located adjacent to parietal cells, which produce histamine, an acid-producing stimulant. Within the antrum and pylorus, pyloric glands contain mucus-secreting cells and endocrine cells, such as G cells which produce gastrin, and D cells which produce somatostatin, an inhibitor of G cell function.

Parietal cell secretion is stimulated by histamine from ECL cells and gastrin from antral G cells. Gastrin also increases acid production by stimulating histamine release from ECL cells. The vagus nerve increases acid production from parietal cells via acetylcholine and via gastrin release. This is the cephalic phase of gastric secretion and precedes the gastric phase which occurs as a result of gastric distension and amino acids in the gastric lumen which stimulate local endocrine production.

Mucosal defence relies upon maintaining a pH gradient between the gastric lumen and epithelium. This is achieved by a mucous barrier which is kept neutral by epithelial bicarbonate secretion. Mucosal blood flow is high which allows rapid removal of acid that does cross the epithelium. Following mucosal injury, repair is rapid and is begun by restitution, which involves cells sliding over the basement membrane to repair epithelial gaps. Cell growth is enhanced following injury and is mediated by trophic factors such as epidermal growth factor (EGF).

DUODENAL ULCER

CLINICAL FEATURES

Patients may describe epigastric pain which is intermittent, particularly occurring at night and partially relieved by food and antacids. Radiation of the pain to the back can occur in posterior duodenal ulcers (DUs). Untreated, the pain persists for a few weeks and usually resolves only to return months later. DU disease cannot be separated from gastric ulcer (GU) and NUD by history; investigation is required to establish the correct diagnosis. Some patients are asymptomatic and only present with the complications of their disease, such as haemorrhage or perforation. Up to 50% of patients will have a family history of DU. Use of NSAIDs is also a predisposing factor.

EPIDEMIOLOGY

The incidence of DU rose steadily until the 1960s but since then has rapidly declined. Peak incidence occurs in the third to fifth decades and is more common in patients with blood group O, particularly those who are non-secretors of the O-related H antigen in mucous glycoprotein. Chronic lung disease, cirrhosis and renal failure are associated with duodenal ulcer but *H. pylori* infection is the commonest association and epidemiological changes in the incidence of DU disease largely reflect the changes in the epidemiology of *H. pylori*.

MANAGEMENT

Diagnosis is usually confirmed by upper GI endoscopy or barium meal studies. Some physicians suggest that in a young patient with dyspeptic symptoms, no sinister features in the history and a positive *H. pylori* serology test, simple *H. pylori* eradication therapy is sufficient without confirmation of DU. In the older age group endoscopy should be performed to confirm the diagnosis and to exclude other important causes of pain such as gastric cancer.

In the last 10 years, treatment of DU has changed. Previously, excellent ulcer-healing rates were achieved with acid suppression therapy alone using H_2-RAs, but relapse rates were high. Following effective *H. pylori* eradication, relapse rates have been drastically cut. In complicated DU such as following severe haemorrhage in the elderly, the risks of re-occurrence should be minimised. This can be best achieved by long-term maintenance therapy with either H_2-RAs or PPIs, which should reduce the recurrence rate to less than 20%.

Surgery was the mainstay for patients with relapsing ulcer disease but is now most frequently employed for complications of DU. Endoscopists frequently encounter patients with post-surgical stomachs and the common operations previously performed are outlined in Figure 1.

COMPLICATIONS

Haemorrhage

Haemorrhage occurs in a small proportion of DUs and is associated with NSAID usage in up to 50% of cases.

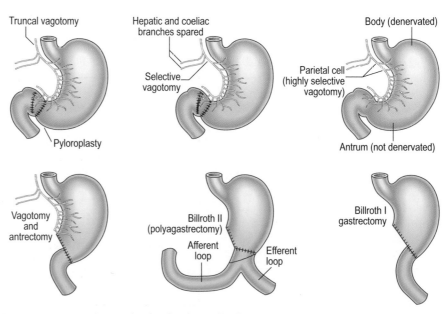

Fig. 1 **Surgical procedures undertaken for ulcers.** (After Rhodes)

Perforation

Perforation complicates DU more frequently than GU and the patient may be asymptomatic prior to the development of an acute abdomen. NSAID use is common. If perforation occurs into surrounding organs, such as the pancreas or omentum, peritonitis may not occur. Conservative management with intravenous hydration, nil by mouth, antibiotics and acid suppression may be used in the very frail, ill or elderly but usually surgery is undertaken to close the perforation. Mortality rises with age and comorbidity.

Gastric outlet obstruction

This usually complicates pyloric canal or duodenal bulb ulcers and occurs in less than 1% of DUs. It results in post-prandial vomiting. There may be an audible succussion splash and it can result in biochemical abnormalities such as hypokalaemia and a metabolic alkalosis. Antral malignancy should be excluded by biopsy. If there is active ulceration, acid suppression therapy alone may be enough for the stenosis to resolve following healing of the ulcer, but chronic ulceration results in fibrotic scarring which requires either endoscopic balloon dilatation or surgery.

Failure to heal

This may occur with patient non-compliance, ineffective *H. pylori* eradication or continued NSAID usage. It is also common amongst smokers and they should be encouraged to stop. Very large DUs may develop in the elderly and require longer courses of treatment.

Resistant ulcers or ulcers present beyond the first part of the duodenum may be due to the rare **Zollinger–Ellison** syndrome. In this condition, islet cell tumours of the pancreas secrete large amounts of gastrin, resulting in an increased parietal cell mass and higher gastric acid output. Consequently multiple or resistant DUs develop. The tumours commonly occur in the head of the pancreas but may also arise in the wall of the duodenum. They are usually small, often multiple and may be difficult to locate. Occurrence may be sporadic or be associated with tumours of the parathyroid and pituitary gland in the autosomal dominant multiple endocrine neoplasia type one syndrome (MEN 1).

The majority of patients have peptic ulcers and a third suffer from diarrhoea. Renal stones may be a complication. A markedly elevated serum gastrin is diagnostic but slightly elevated levels can be difficult to interpret and secretion stimulation tests are required. Hypo- or achlorhydria, caused by acid suppression therapy or pernicious anaemia, leads to a rise in serum gastrin which may confuse interpretation and so acid suppression therapy should be discontinued at least 3 weeks prior to testing. Surgical resection following localisation in the absence of metastases offers the best chance of cure. Tumours may be localised by endoscopic ultrasound, CT, angiography or octreotide scanning. Acid suppression with high doses of PPIs may be used to treat the peptic ulceration.

GASTRIC ULCER

CLINICAL FEATURES

Presentation is more variable than with DU. Patients may present with epigastric pain relieved or aggravated by eating, but often symptoms are vague, with anorexia, post-prandial fullness and weight loss. GU should be considered in the elderly presenting with these symptoms. Anaemia is also commonly found as GUs frequently bleed.

EPIDEMIOLOGY

In the last century, gastric ulcers were much more common than now and affected a younger age group. During this century, this has changed and GUs have a peak age incidence 10 years higher than DUs, occurring most frequently in the sixth and seventh decades. *H. pylori* and NSAID usage are frequent associations, the latter particularly in elderly women. Acute ulcers may be induced by medical stress such as following severe burns or neurosurgery. Benign ulcers most frequently occur on the lesser curve whilst those occurring on the greater curve or in the fundus of the stomach are more likely to be malignant. Pre-pyloric ulcers are associated with elevated gastric acid production and behave like DUs.

MANAGEMENT

Diagnosis is best confirmed by endoscopy as GUs shown by barium studies require endoscopy to exclude malignancy. All GUs require multiple biopsy from both the rim and crater of the ulcer. Treatment is longer than for DUs and unlike DUs, healing has to be confirmed by repeat endoscopy and biopsy usually performed after 6 weeks of treatment, as failure to heal may signify malignancy. Care has to be taken at endoscopy as previous or current PPI usage can lead to re-epithelialisation, even over malignant ulcers and their presence can be missed.

Treatment is with a PPI for 6 weeks or more. *H. pylori* should be eradicated when found and NSAIDs and smoking discontinued. Treatment failure following 12–16 weeks' treatment may be an indication for surgery, particularly as malignancy may be missed despite multiple biopsies. Similar complications to those of DU may occur and are treated in the same way. Following *H. pylori* eradication and withdrawal of NSAIDs, GUs are unlikely to recur but if they do, maintenance PPI therapy is appropriate.

Peptic ulcer disease

- Parietal cells in the stomach produce acid and are controlled by histamine and gastrin.
- Mucosal defence relies upon maintaining an alkaline mucous barrier and a high mucosal blood flow to rapidly remove hydrogen ions that cross the mucus barrier.
- Duodenal and gastric ulcers are strongly associated with *H. pylori* infection and treatment is directed at eradicating the infection in addition to acid suppression.
- Non-*H. pylori*-associated ulcers may be caused by aspirin or NSAID usage, hypercalcaemia, physiological stress or Zollinger–Ellison syndrome.
- Gastric ulcers have a malignant potential and should always be biopsied at endoscopy, and healing confirmed following treatment.
- Proton pump inhibitors may mask malignant gastric ulcers, so endoscopy is best performed when this medication has ceased.

GASTRIC TUMOURS

MALIGNANT

GASTRIC CANCER

Clinical features

In its early stages, gastric cancer is usually asymptomatic and consequently patients frequently present late. Early gastric cancer is usually only detected by screening which is undertaken in areas with a high incidence such as Japan. Perhaps as a result of inexperience of endoscopists in the West and widespread use of PPIs prior to endoscopy, early gastric cancer is often missed. As the disease progresses, epigastric pain and weight loss or gastric outflow obstruction are frequent presenting symptoms. There is a slight male predominance (1.7:1) and peak occurrence is in the seventh decade in the low-incidence areas and 10 years younger where the incidence is higher.

Epidemiology

In the USA it is the eleventh commonest cancer but may be the second commonest worldwide. There is great geographical variation with a greater than ten-fold variation in incidence between low areas such as the USA and Europe, and high areas as such as Japan, China and Russia.

Table 1 **TNM staging of gastric cancer**

T1 Confined to mucosa or submucosa					
T2 Muscularis propria involved					
T3 Serosal surface involved					
T4 Adjacent organs involved					

N represents extent of node involvement

N0	No lymph node involvement
N1	Perigastric nodes within 3 cm of primary
N2	More distant perigastric and regional nodes
N3	More distant intra-abdominal nodes

M represents presence or absence of metastases

M0	No metastases
M1	Distant metastases

Staging using the TNM classification

	N0	N1	N2	N3	M1
T1	IA	IB	II	IV	IV
T2	IB	II	IIIA	IV	IV
T3	II	IIIA	IIIB	IV	IV
T4	IIIA	IIIB	IV	IV	IV

STAGE	5-year survival
IA	95%
IB	82%
II	55%
IIIA	30%
IIIB	15%
IV	2%

This is probably due to environmental factors as when populations move from high- to low-rate areas the incidence falls rapidly. Environmental factors that appear to be important are:

- *H. pylori*
- low socio-economic class
- high dietary intake of salted, pickled and smoked foods
- low intake of vitamin C, fruit and vegetables.

Predisposing conditions include Barrett's oesophagus which is associated with cancer of the cardia, pernicious anaemia, gastric atrophy and intestinal metaplasia, post-gastrectomy (particularly after 20 years) adenomas and familial adenomatous polyposis.

Two histological types are described:

1. an **intestinal type** shows more differentiation with glandular formation and it is the variation in the incidence of this cancer worldwide which accounts for the differences.
2. a **diffuse type** shows less differentiation with sheets of invasive cells, without glands, occasionally with mucin-producing signet ring cells. The prevalence of this cancer worldwide is similar.

Management

Diagnosis depends on endoscopy and biopsy. Cancers have different endoscopic appearances and may be GU-like with features that suggest malignancy (such as rolled or irregular edges). However these are unreliable features and histology is essential. There may be diffuse infiltration by malignant cells which gives the gastric mucosa a thickened appearance – linitis plastica – or tumours may be polypoid or proliferative. Early gastric cancer (defined as not penetrating the submucosa) may be more difficult to detect at endoscopy as mucosal lesions may be minor and this underlines the necessity for biopsy of abnormal looking areas of mucosa.

Japan has pioneered the detection of early gastric cancer and has shown that early surgery substantially increases survival. However, gastric cancer has an incidence in excess of 100 per 100 000 and these programmes have not been successfully exported to areas with lower incidence. Even where recognised premalignant conditions such as intestinal metaplasia are discovered, there is no evidence that screening is useful.

Surgery offers the only hope of cure and following the detection of cancer, preoperative staging is undertaken. CT scanning can detect enlarged lymph nodes which, if greater than 1 cm in size, suggest metastatic infiltration, and can assist the assessment of local and distal spread (Fig. 1). Transabdominal ultrasound is readily available but it only visualises local lymph nodes if they are markedly enlarged. Endoscopic ultrasound is much less widely available and interpretation is difficult, but it allows assessment of both the depth of mucosal penetration of the tumour and local involvement of lymph nodes. This method will increase in use as it becomes more widely available.

Radical surgery with extensive lymph node clearance appears to lead to improved survival. In advanced tumours with gastric outflow obstruction, palliative surgery in the form of a gastroenterostomy may be performed. Survival progressively deteriorates with more advanced tumours (Table 1). In patients who are unfit or decline surgery, treatment can be directed at the complications of the tumour – patients often develop recurrent anaemia which can be treated endoscopically by coagulation of the tumour surface with either laser or argon beam photocoagulation and blood transfusion. Gastric outflow obstruction may be prevented with repeated laser or argon beam treatment to maintain a patent channel but often the repeated sessions are more arduous for the patient than the single, surgical fashioning of a gastroenterostomy. As in all patients with terminal disease close involvement with a palliative care team should be sought at an early stage.

There is growing interest in the use of chemotherapy either postoperatively or more recently preoperatively (neoadjuvant chemotherapy) in an attempt to increase survival. Long-term results of these treatments are awaited.

Complications of previous gastric surgery

Before effective medical treatment for ulcer disease, gastric surgery was widely performed for benign conditions, but is now most commonly performed for cancer. Various procedures were performed which are still encountered at endoscopy. Some of the more common complications of gastric surgery are:

• **Diarrhoea.** This can be due to rapid gastric emptying, small bowel bacterial overgrowth or bile salt diarrhoea. It may respond to small meals, antibiotics in the presence of bacterial overgrowth or cholestyramine.

• **Vomiting.** This may resolve gradually postoperatively, but where there is persistent vomiting, several causes should be considered. Biliary reflux gastritis is very common post-resection, and promotility agents or chelating agents such as cholestyramine and aluminium hydroxide should be tried. Stomal ulcers can occur and require acid suppression therapy. Delayed gastric emptying may respond to promotility agents.

• **Early dumping.** Patients experience abdominal fullness and faintness a few minutes after eating. There may be transient hypotension and hypokalaemia. The mechanism is unclear but small, more frequent meals may be helpful. Guar gum and somatostatin may be used and surgical revision is sometimes undertaken but with limited success.

• **Late dumping.** Hypoglycaemia occurs 2–3 hours after eating and faintness is experienced. A glucose tolerance test reveals an early rise to an elevated blood glucose at the time of the meal with subsequent hypoglycaemia at the time of symptoms. Small meals and guar gum may help, as may acarbose, a new agent, which results in gradual carbohydrate absorption along the small bowel achieving a less severe early rise and subsequent fall in blood glucose level.

• **Weight loss.** Reduced intake owing to early satiety, recurrence of malignant disease and small bowel bacterial overgrowth may all be responsible.

• **Anaemia.** Iron deficiency is the commonest anaemia to occur after gastric resection and may occur many years after surgery. It is probably caused by decreased absorption resulting from decreased gastric acidity and vitamin C which facilitates iron absorption.

Lower GI causes of blood loss need to be considered and excluded as should stomal ulceration or recurrence of previous gastric cancer. Vitamin B_{12} deficiency can occur as a result of lack of intrinsic factor or bacterial overgrowth.

Rarer complications

Afferent loop syndrome is where a poorly draining afferent loop following a polya gastrectomy distends with bile during a meal causing pain and then suddenly empties resulting in bilious vomiting. Surgical refashioning may be necessary.

If recurrent ulceration occurs following antrectomy then incomplete excision and **retained antrum** may be the cause but Zollinger–Ellison syndrome should also be considered.

Post-vagotomy dysphagia is usually transient and is thought to be related to local trauma and oedema.

LYMPHOMA

This is the second most common gastric malignancy and represents just 5% of the total. Primary gastric lymphomas have a similar presentation and appearance to adeno-carcinoma and are usually B cell type. There is a strong association with *H. pylori* and early MALT lymphoma may regress following *H. pylori* eradication therapy. More advanced disease requires surgery and chemotherapy. Patients with AIDS also have an increased risk of gastric lymphoma.

BENIGN

GASTRIC POLYPS

These are relatively unusual, frequently small and rarely of clinical significance. Larger polyps may be adenomatous and should be snared if possible, but small polyps are usually hyperplastic and do not require excision.

LEIOMYOMAS

These are an occasional cause of upper GI haemorrhage. They have a characteristic endoscopic and radiographic appearance with an ulcer crater occurring at the apex of the polyp. They can attain a considerable size and larger lesions have a higher risk of malignancy. They are dumb-bell shaped and are not usually amenable to endoscopic treatment but require surgical excision.

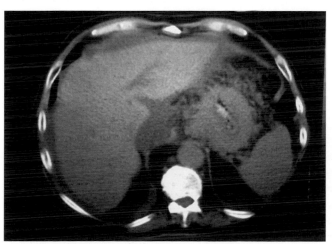

Fig. 1 **CT scan showing thickened gastric wall in a gastric cancer.**

Gastric tumours

• Gastric cancers frequently present late in their natural history and screening is only feasible in areas of high incidence.
• Predisposing factors for gastric cancer include *H. pylori*, pernicious anaemia, gastric atrophy, previous gastric surgery and familial adenomatous polyposis.
• Surgery offers the only hope of cure and survival is closely correlated with disease stage at diagnosis.
• Before effective medical treatment, gastric surgery was frequently performed for benign disease and complications include diarrhoea, vomiting, dumping, weight loss and anaemia.

GALLSTONES

CLINICAL FEATURES

Half of patients with gallstones experience no problems but 35% of patients with gallstones discovered by chance will require treatment over the next 10 years as a result of either pain or complications. A number of clinical conditions may develop as a result of gallstones depending upon their location (Fig. 1) .

Acute cholecystitis

The abrupt onset of severe, right upper quadrant (RUQ) pain, which is constant and does not remit, points to acute cholecystitis. It is usually accompanied by pyrexia and leucocytosis and is a result of impaction of a gallstone in the cystic duct with associated infection in 50% of cases. Jaundice may develop if there is compression of the common bile duct (CBD) either because of the stone in the cystic duct or as result of surrounding inflammation (Mirizzi's syndrome). In seriously ill, elderly patients a similar picture may develop in the absence of gallstones and is termed acute acalculous cholecystitis and carries a poor prognosis.

Biliary pain / chronic cholecystitis

The symptoms are of intermittent, dull RUQ pain – constant or colicky. It may occur at any time and is not necessarily related to meals. It resolves spontaneously within a few hours and is not associated with systemic upset. These symptoms are a common indication for cholecystectomy, but it is difficult to determine that patients' symptoms are caused by their gallstones in this group. Symptoms of non-specific, post-prandial pain, bloating and fatty food intolerance are not good discriminators and 25% of patients who undergo cholecystectomy for these symptoms will experience continued discomfort postoperatively.

Choledocholithiasis

Stones which have migrated into or formed within the CBD may be asymptomatic and be discovered by an elevation in the alkaline phosphatase level. They are usually associated with biliary type pain and intermittent jaundice and can cause obstruction. Removal of these stones is essential as there is a high complication rate (Table 3).

Cholangitis

This occurs when there is infection in the biliary tree, usually as a result of CBD stones. Patients present with biliary pain, jaundice, fever and often rigors. The septicaemia is usually due to Gram-negative organisms, is frequently severe and may be life-threatening.

Less common complications

As stones pass the ampulla of Vater, they can induce a biliary pancreatitis. Stones may erode through the gallbladder wall into the ileum causing a cholecystenteric fistula. Gallbladder stones may be associated with calcification of the gallbladder wall ('porcelain' gallbladder), which carries a 20% risk of developing gallbladder cancer. Chronic cholelithiasis alone carries an increased but much lower risk of developing cancer.

AETIOLOGY

Bile is a super-saturated solution of cholesterol. Cholesterol does not crystallise out because of a combination of factors including :

1. the detergent activity of bile salts (paradoxically produced from cholesterol) and the polar lipid lecithin
2. gallbladder motility.

Gallstones develop when these mechanisms fail and there is an originating nidus for stone formation which is often mucin or bacteria.

80% of gallstones are cholesterol or mixed cholesterol stones where cholesterol is the major constituent. Pigment stones form the bulk of the rest and comprise predominantly bile pigment and are most common in chronic haemolytic states (Table 1).

EPIDEMIOLOGY

Incidence varies with age: 5% at age 20, rising to 30% over 50. There is a 2:1 predominance in females. There are wide ethnic variations with American Pima Indians having an incidence of 70% in females aged 20. Scandinavia also has high incidences

Table 1 **Types of gallstones**

Stone type	Predisposing factors
Cholesterol	Obesity, diabetes mellitus, multiparity, terminal ileal disease, hyperlipidaemia, oestrogens/oral contraceptive pill, total parenteral nutrition
Black/pigment	Haemolysis, cirrhosis

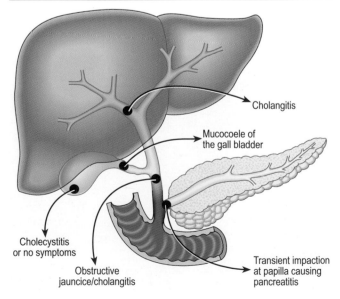

Fig. 1 **Gallstones and the conditions they cause.** (After Rhodes)

Table 2 **Conditions resulting from gallstones**

	Chronic cholecystitis	Acute cholecystitis	Choledocholithiasis	Cholangitis
Clinical picture	Poorly localised pain Remits spontaneously in hours Local tenderness Apyrexial	Severe RUQ pain Severe tenderness Pyrexia	Intermittent jaundice Intermittent colic Pyrexia suggests cholangitis	Rigors RUQ pain Pyrexia
Laboratory findings	Usually normal	Leucocytosis Mild AP elevation	Elevated AP & bilirubin	Elevated AP & bilirubin
Diagnostic test	Ultrasonography Oral cholecystography	Ultrasonography	ERCP Ultrasonography	ERCP Ultrasonography

AP = alkaline phosphatase; RUQ = right upper quadrant

excreted in the bile, subsequently being concentrated in the gallbladder. This shows gallstones as filling defects within the gallbladder and demonstrates that the cystic duct is not obstructed. Following a fatty meal, the ability of the gallbladder to contract can also be measured. A functioning gallbladder and a non-obstructed, cystic duct are prerequisites for consideration of bile dissolution therapy.

Endoscopic retrograde cholangiopancreatography (ERCP) is the technique of choice to demonstrate CBD stones as it also allows therapeutic interventions at the same time.

Computerised tomography (CT) is not particularly helpful in gallstone disease but fine slice images may demonstrate CBD stones not seen at ultrasound. MR cholangiography is in its infancy and its place in hepatobiliary disease is being defined.

TREATMENT

Cholecystitis

Acute cholecystitis requires analgesia, intravenous support and antibiotics, and usually settles with these measures. Subsequent cholecystectomy may then be performed when the acute episode has resolved.

Careful selection of patients with chronic cholecystitis is important as not all patients are pain-free when the gallbladder is removed; symptoms may abate spontaneously and not recur; and there is an increasing, associated, operative mortality with advancing age.

Laparoscopic cholecystectomy has increased the acceptability of the procedure for patients and has consequently become widely available. There appears to be an increased risk of bile duct injury at the time of the procedure, particularly when carried out by inexperienced surgeons. However, the replacement of a large subcostal scar with three porthole incisions reduces postoperative pain and hospital stay from 10 to less than 3 days.

Cholangitis

Acute cholangitis is a serious infection which may be life-threatening. Antibiotics such as third generation cephalosporins or amino-quinolones should be used. Careful attention should be paid to fluid balance, urine output and renal function. Cholangitis is usually caused by CBD stones and therefore ERCP is required early in its management, to allow confirmation of biliary stones and their extraction.

Following sphincterotomy, the bile duct can be trawled with either an inflatable balloon or a basket to extract the stones. If it is not possible to clear the duct, then an endoscopic stent may be inserted to facilitate bile drainage and reduce the risk of further episodes of cholangitis. Subsequent attempts may be made to clear the bile duct or in the elderly these stents may be left in place. As long-term stents can occlude and further episodes of cholangitis can occur, stent replacement may be necessary.

Postcholecystectomy pain

Following cholecystectomy, some patients continue to experience symptoms such as bloating, fatty food intolerance and dyspepsia. These symptoms usually predated the surgery and are often due to the irritable bowel syndrome. There is also a group of patients who have convincing biliary pain after stones have been removed. Liver function tests may be abnormal and some patients may be jaundiced. ERCP shows a dilated CBD without stones and there may be delayed excretion of contrast medium. This points towards sphincter of Oddi dysfunction which in more severe cases may benefit from endoscopic sphincterotomy.

Medical management of gallbladder stones

Dissolution therapy can be considered in patients with uncomplicated gallstone disease who are unwilling or unfit for surgery. The prerequisites for treatment are that the stones should be non-calcified, the gallbladder should be functioning and the cystic duct not obstructed. The bile acids, chenodeoxycholic acid and ursodeoxycholic acid are available and need to be given for long periods to be successful. They have no effect on pigment stones.

Gallstones

- Gallstones are common and many are asymptomatic. Patients may have abdominal pain caused by their gallstones, so patient selection for cholecystectomy is very important.
- Conditions caused by gallstones vary depending on the location of the stones.
- Cholangitis is a severe infection which should be recognised early and treated aggressively.
- Ultrasound is good at detecting gallbladder stones but not CBD stones. However, CBD or hepatic duct dilatation implies obstruction.
- Ideally, CBD stones should be cleared but long-term endoprosthetic stenting is acceptable in the elderly.
- Laparoscopic cholecystectomy carries an increased risk of bile duct injury but is highly acceptable to patients, as it means less postoperative pain and shorter hospital stays.

IRRITABLE BOWEL SYNDROME

EPIDEMIOLOGY

The symptoms associated with irritable bowel syndrome (IBS) are experienced by up to 20% of the population in the West. Although most sufferers will not consult a doctor, the condition still represents 50% of referrals to gastroenterologists. It is a transcultural condition and and is recognised in Africa, India and China. It is more common in urban populations, and is twice as prevalent in women. Symptoms tend to begin in the teens and twenties and decrease with age but the condition may be lifelong.

CLINICAL FEATURES (Fig. 1)

There is a host of symptoms that are associated with IBS but the following are the most important.

Abdominal pain

This is the central feature and is usually described as colicky or constant, particularly in the lower abdomen or left iliac fossa. However, the pain may take on a variety of qualities and may be located anywhere within the abdomen. The intensity of the pain varies from intermittently, mildly annoying to extremely severe. It may be present at any time of day or night but it is unlikely to awaken sufferers from their sleep. It is frequently worsened by eating and relieved by defaecation.

Altered bowel habit

It is worth remembering that the range of normality for defaecation is between once every 3 days and three times a day.

The bowel habit in IBS is most often alternating in that sufferers describe periods of infrequent, hard often 'pellet-like' motions interspersed with increased frequency of looser stools. It is usually possible to determine a diarrhoea-or constipation-predominant IBS type, which has implications for treatment strategies. There is often urgency, a feeling of incomplete evacuation and passage of mucus associated with defaecation. Rectal bleeding, steatorrhoea and nocturnal defaecation are not features of IBS and warrant further investigation. Passage of mucus is often described as being increased by sufferers but a mechanism for this has not been found nor has it been reliably documented.

Bloating

A sensation of abdominal distension is often described although it is quite difficult to demonstrate this consistently in IBS sufferers. Younger women report that they feel as if they are 9 months pregnant. This symptom may be the result of increased intestinal gas, which is probably swallowed air, but may also reflect altered intestinal motility.

Non-colonic gastrointestinal symptoms

Frequent associated symptoms are of heartburn, nausea, postprandial fullness and pain which may be attributable to the gallbladder or biliary tree. This may be due to a generalized smooth muscle abnormality.

Extra-intestinal symptoms

These include urinary frequency and dysuria. Dyspareunia may be present if specifically enquired about, and there may be fea-

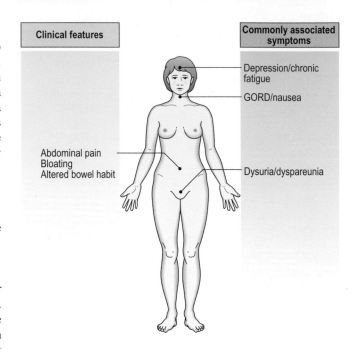

Fig. 1 **Clinical features of IBS.**

tures of fibromyalgia or chronic fatigue syndrome. Psychological factors may be relevant as there does appear to be an increased incidence of depressive illness and neuroticism amongst sufferers.

In order to try to standardise the diagnosis, first Manning in 1978 described a series of symptoms which positively discriminated for IBS and subsequently in Rome these symptoms were refined (Table 1). However, these symptoms commonly occur in other organic gut conditions.

PATHOPHYSIOLOGY

Perhaps because of the heterogeneous nature of the condition and lack of a definitive diagnostic test, elucidating the cause or causes of symptoms has been unsuccessful. Although no single, consistent feature has been identified, abnormalities have been detected in:
- **gastrointestinal motility** – there are shorter transit times and hypomotility in diarrhoea-predominant IBS, and reduced, high amplitude, peristaltic contractions in constipation-predominant IBS. The observed motility changes, however, do not correlate well with clinical features.
- **altered visceral sensation** – increased sensitivity to

Table 1 **Rome criteria for the diagnosis of IBS**

At least 3 months of continuous or recurrent symptoms of:

1 Abdominal pain or discomfort that is:
- relieved with defaecation and/or
- associated with a change in stool frequency and/or
- associated with a change in stool consistency

2 Two or more of the following at least on a quarter of days or occasions:
- altered stool frequency
- altered stool form
- altered stool passage (straining, urgency, incomplete evacuation)
- passage of mucus
- bloating or feeling of abdominal distension

inflated balloons in both small and large bowel has been demonstrated and increased rectal sensitivity is a common finding.

- **psychological abnormalities** – both sufferers and doctors recognise the effect of psychological stress on the symptoms, but quantifying this is difficult. Psychological symptoms are more prevalent in IBS sufferers, particularly in those referred to hospital and up to 60% may fulfil diagnostic criteria for mental disorders such as depression and anxiety.

Disease phobia and bodily preoccupation are also more common. Some patients describe the onset of their symptoms following an episode of gastroenteritis and there does not appear to be a major psychological component to their condition.

- **endocrine changes** – many women recognise that the symptoms of IBS are more marked during menstruation. No obvious hormonal correlations have been made but there are increased levels of prostaglandin E_2 and F_2 around this time and this may be important. Symptoms often worsen following hysterectomy which is presumably not explained by hormonal changes but may be due to damage to pelvic nerves at the time of surgery. Unfortunately, some patients undergo hysterectomy when the pain is actually caused by IBS which persists after the operation – a problem that needs to be recognised by gynaecologists.

MANAGEMENT

A thorough history is of prime importance because of the lack of a diagnostic test and broad differential diagnosis that the symptoms of IBS create. It was formerly taught that the diagnosis should be made positively and not by excluding other conditions, but some diagnoses are excluded by the history and examination and others excluded by simple tests. During the history-taking, special attention should be given to ensure that sinister symptoms such as marked weight loss, rectal bleeding, steatorrhoea, nocturnal diarrhoea, and associated skin or joint symptoms are not present.

In addition to a general examination, sigmoidoscopy should be carried out and a rectal biopsy taken, particularly in diarrhoea-predominant IBS. Blood investigations should include full blood count, biochemistry, liver function tests, and the inflammatory markers: erythrocyte sedimentation rate (ESR) and C-reactive protein (CRP).

With a good history and a normal result from the above investigations, a positive diagnosis of IBS can be made, particularly in the younger age group (<40 years). It is prudent to include further colonic examination such as barium enema studies in the older age group to exclude colonic neoplasia.

Over-investigation may simply serve to convince sufferers that the physician is not sure of the diagnosis and is best avoided. Occasionally, factors will confound the diagnosis such as a slightly raised CRP which will usually warrant further GI investigations but may be due to many non-GI conditions.

TREATMENT

Successful treatment of sufferers with IBS takes considerable skill on the part of the physician. The approach taken at the time of diagnosis will have long-term effects on how patients view their condition. Careful discussion of possible mechanisms of the causes of pain and relevant trigger factors such as diet and anxiety and the universal nature of the condition will often serve to reassure sufferers.

THERAPEUTIC OPTIONS

Dietary manipulation

An increase in dietary fibre has been favoured advice for years but makes as many sufferers worse as it does better. It is most useful in constipation-predominant IBS but may worsen bloating. Exclusion diets whereby various food types are removed then subsequently reintroduced into the diet until triggers are found may be beneficial in some cases but are a protracted and rather arduous treatment. Lactose intolerance may affect 10% of the population and contribute to symptoms of diarrhoea and bloating. Exclusion of dairy products from the diet is probably the easiest way to confirm this although a lactose breath test can also be used. Patients will often experiment with their diet themselves and may try unsubstantiated protocols such as low yeast diets which will usually do no harm.

Drugs

Anticholinergics such as dicyclomine and hyoscine may help pain and diarrhoea but can have side-effects with urinary retention and effects on intraocular pressures.

Antispasmodics such as mebeverine and peppermint-based products (particularly for constipation-dominant IBS) may help pain and bloating and are widely used as they do not have anticholinergic side-effects.

Antidepressants have long been used in patients with severe IBS and it may be most appropriate to consider a tricyclic for diarrhoea-predominant IBS and a selective serotonin reuptake inhibitor for constipation-predominant IBS.

Prokinetics may help post-prandial fullness, bloating and constipation but worsen diarrhoea-predominant IBS.

If constipation does not respond to adequate bulking of the stool or an osmotic laxative then a stimulant laxative may be required. Likewise, only if diarrhoea is intractable and troublesome should constipating agents such as loperamide be used.

Complementary therapies

Hypnotherapy, stress management, psychotherapy and acupuncture have all been used and may help some sufferers.

Irritable bowel syndrome

- Irritable bowel syndrome is the commonest condition seen by gastroenterologists and one of the commonest in general practice.
- In patients under 40 years, history, examination including sigmoidoscopy and simple blood test should be sufficient to reach a diagnosis, but over age 40 it is sensible to include a barium enema as part of the investigation.
- Many other extra-colonic symptoms may occur as part of the syndrome.
- Effective management includes taking time to discuss the condition with patients at the time of diagnosis.
- Reassurance, dietary advice and drugs may all be used to treat sufferers and requirements may change with time.

CHRONIC PANCREATITIS

CLINICAL FEATURES

The three important features of chronic pancreatitis are pain, steatorrhoea resulting from exocrine dysfunction and diabetes mellitus resulting from endocrine dysfunction.

Pain. The pain is usually located in the upper abdomen but is poorly localised. It is described as a boring, deep pain which may radiate to the back and is worsened after meals. It may be nocturnal. Its severity is not proportional to steatorrhoea and correlates poorly with loss of exocrine function or structural abnormality. The pain is the most difficult problem to treat and can be frustrating for both the patient and the physician.

Steatorrhoea. Lipase secretion has to be reduced to less than 10% of normal for steatorrhoea to develop and consequently this is a symptom which develops when the disease is advanced. Fat-soluble vitamins (A, D, E and K) are rarely sufficiently malabsorbed to cause symptoms. Stools are passed 2–3 times per day, are pale and may contain droplets of oil.

Diabetes. For overt diabetes to develop, more than 80% of the gland needs to be affected, which means that diabetes is also usually a late complication. However, abnormalities in the glucose tolerance test are detectable much earlier.

The vast majority of patients will describe a heavy, sustained alcohol drinking habit and only rarely will there be a significant family history or associated medical history.

Examination is usually normal although a mass may be palpable when a pseudocyst or cancer has developed. The spleen may be enlarged when the splenic vein has thrombosed.

PATHOPHYSIOLOGY

Aetiology

Alcohol is the major cause and the history is usually of > 150 g/day for more than 5 years. Less than 20% of heavy drinkers develop chronic pancreatitis and it is unclear why this is so, but there may be a diet rich in fat in those that do develop chronic pancreatitis. A preceding history of recurrent episodes of acute pancreatitis is not usually present.

A tropical form of the disease is described which may be associated with protein malnutrition and intraductal stones.

Familial and other inherited causes also occur (Table 1) although in up to 30%, the cause is obscure.

It is unclear what initiates and perpetuates the chronic inflammation and fibrosis that develop within the pancreas. One theory is that a diet rich in lipid increases protein secretion by the pancreas. This may cause precipitation of these proteins in pancreatic ducts resulting in partial obstruction, which, when associated with toxic metabolites from alcohol, initiates the process. Another proposal is that chronic pancreatitis is a result of recurrent episodes of acute pancreatitis.

Classification

Three groups have been described:

1. **chronic calcified pancreatitis** – fibrosis, intraductal protein plugs and stones result in ductal injury; alcohol is the major cause.
2. **chronic obstructive pancreatitis** – obstruction of the main duct with proximal, uniform, ductal dilatation and subsequent atrophy and fibrosis; this is much less common and is due to either an intraductal tumour or a stricture.
3. **chronic inflammatory pancreatitis** – fibrosis and a mononuclear infiltrate associated with conditions such as Sjögren's syndrome and primary sclerosing cholangitis.

MANAGEMENT

Diagnosis

The triad of pain, steatorrhoea and diabetes is unlikely to occur until late in the disease and patients more usually present with pain. There may be no signs of chronic liver disease as this too only develops in one-fifth of heavy drinkers.

Simple blood tests are not usually helpful although there may be diabetes or at least an impaired glucose tolerance test. Serum lipase and amylase elevation is unusual and only tends to occur if the pancreatic duct is blocked or there is a pseudocyst. An obstructive pattern in the liver profile may occur if stricturing of the CBD has developed.

The important differential diagnoses include peptic ulcer, biliary tract disease, mesenteric ischaemia and gastric or pancreatic malignancy, and appropriate investigation is necessary to exclude these.

Pancreatic function tests

A number of tests are available to assess endocrine pancreatic function. Some tests quantify enzyme production, measured

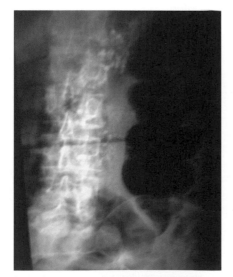

Fig. 1 **Plain X-ray of abdomen showing calcific pancreatitis.**

Table 2 **Tests of exocrine pancreatic function**

Test	Comments
Hormone stimulation test	Secretin stimulates bicarbonate production. CCK stimulates enzyme production Duodenal intubation necessary. Most sensitive and specific (S/S)
Bentiromide test	Synthetic peptide cleaved by chymotrypsin, to produce PABA. Metabolic product measured in urine. Moderate S/S
Pancreolauryl test	Fluorescein dilaurate hydrolysed by elastase. Fluorescein measured in urine Similar S/S to bentiromide test
Faecal chymotrypsin	Pancreatic secretion of proteases. Faecal measurement
Faecal fat	Reduction of pancreatic lipase results in maldigestion of fat Does not distinguish from malabsorption

following intubation of the duodenum and stimulation of the pancreas either by hormones or a test meal, while other tests quantify production of metabolites of reactions catalysed by pancreatic enzymes (Table 2). As a group, the tests have similar drawbacks in that they require accurate intubation of the duodenum and all depend on complete sample collection. The other major drawback is that a significantly abnormal test frequently does not develop until late in the condition when diagnostic uncertainty is often much less. They are of no use in monitoring the condition.

Imaging

Various imaging modalities are used, often in combination. **Plain abdominal X-ray** reveals pancreatic calcification or stones in up to two-thirds of patients. It may be necessary to perform a lateral X-ray as vertebrae may obscure the view (Fig. 1). **Transabdominal ultrasound** has the drawback that overlying bowel may obscure the view obtained, but it is moderately sensitive at detecting abnormalities of texture of the pancreas, variations in ductal calibre and pseudocysts. **Endoscopic ultrasound** overcomes some of the visualisation problems and is probably more sensitive and specific. **CT** has a sensitivity of up to 90% and specificity of the same order. It will detect variation in ductal diameter, and ectatic side branches, changes in the parenchyma, calcification and complications of chronic pancreatitis such as pseudocyst formation (Fig. 2). **Endoscopic retrograde cholangiopancreatography (ERCP)** is probably the most sensitive imaging technique (Fig. 3) but

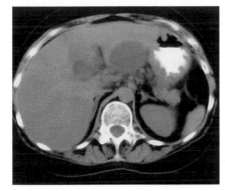

Fig. 2 **CT scan with central pseudocyst.**

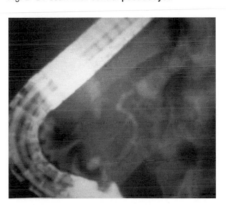

Fig. 3 **ERCP of chronic pancreatitis with distortion of the pancreatic duct.**

still fails to correlate with functional tests in around 25% of cases.

TREATMENT

It is important to try to minimise disease progression and this is best done by total alcohol avoidance particularly in those in whom alcohol is the cause.

Pain

Analgesia requirement should be titrated against need but often spirals upwards to considerable opiate requirement and subsequent addiction. Care should be taken in controlling associated side-effects such as constipation which can lead to abdominal pain inappropriately attributed to the pancreas. Pancreatic enzyme supplemen-

tation is usually used and may be helpful as may an anti-oxidant cocktail given daily. Coeliac axis nerve block may lead to temporary improvement in pain but frequently symptoms recur. Surgery including partial resections and drainage procedures may be helpful in the most severe cases but it is difficult to obtain controlled data for these procedures. Resection of tissue including endocrine cells results in brittle diabetes which is difficult to manage.

Steatorrhoea

Dietary enzyme supplementation usually controls this. Lipase inactivation by gastric acid may result in more than the expected 30 000 units of lipase per meal estimated to be required to prevent steatorrhoea. Gelatin capsules and acid suppression therapy may help.

Diabetes

This is often brittle and wide fluctuations in blood glucose are seen with exogenous insulin.

Complications

Pseudocysts may occur in up to 25% of patients with chronic pancreatitis and if they are of significant size require drainage either surgically or endoscopically. Bleeding may occur into a pseudocyst or there may be erosion into surrounding vessels. Splenic vein thrombosis may occur resulting in gastric and oesophageal varices. Pancreatic cancer is more common in patients with chronic pancreatitis and represents the major differential diagnosis when obstructive jaundice occurs with a stricture of the CBD. Differentiation between the two conditions is difficult and serum markers (CA 19-9), CT and biopsy may all be necessary to confirm the diagnosis.

Table 1 **Causes of chronic pancreatitis**

Alcohol	150 g/day for prolonged periods
Cystic fibrosis	Autosomal recessive. 1:2000 births amongst Caucasians
Tropical	The young, near the equator. Intraductal calculi. Aetiology unknown
Hereditary	The young, pancreatic calcification. Aetiology unknown
Obstructive	Chronic obstruction, possibly owing to pancreas divisum/acquired obstruction
Idiopathic	Up to 30% cause unknown
Alpha-₁ antitrypsin deficiency	Usually asymptomatic pancreatic insufficiency
Haemochromatosis	Usually asymptomatic pancreatic insufficiency
Hypertriglyceridaemia	

Chronic pancreatitis

- Pain, steatorrhoea and diabetes mellitus are the main clinical features of chronic pancreatitis of which pain is usually the most troublesome.
- Severe exocrine and endocrine dysfunction are necessary to produce steatorrhoea and diabetes mellitus.
- Alcohol is by far the commonest aetiological agent.
- A combination of tests including functional and anatomical assessment may be necessary.
- Pain can be difficult to control and opiate addiction is not uncommon, but may be helped by pancreatic enzymes and anti-oxidants.

THE CLINICAL APPROACH

HISTORY

Patients with acute abdominal pain are usually first seen at an accident and emergency department and present a considerable challenge to the junior doctor. A consistent, structured approach is necessary to avoid missing diagnoses by not considering them. The artificial separation of patients into 'medical' and 'surgical' categories is not helpful diagnostically and both physicians and surgeons have to be alert to conditions that they would not normally treat.

Localisation

The site of pain must be established first and it should be remembered that visceral pain is poorly localised but pain caused by peritonitis is more accurately described. Anatomical location is the first clue to the diagnosis (Fig. 1).

Associated symptoms

Associated symptoms help to focus on the system or organ causing the pain. Respiratory symptoms point to basal pneumonia causing diaphragmatic irritation. Nausea and vomiting are signs of an upper GI cause, whereas jaundice or rigors implicate the biliary tree. A previous change in bowel habit, blood loss per rectum or intermittent left iliac fossa pain suggests the colon. Dysuria or haematuria indicates a renal cause, particularly if pain is referred from the loin to the pelvis, whilst a history of poor urinary stream and dribbling in an elderly man suggests acute urinary outflow obstruction. A careful gynaecological history is necessary and pregnancy should be considered in all women – even when it is felt to be 'impossible' by the patient.

Previous history

Previous diagnoses should be elucidated and particularly previous surgery as this predisposes to the development of adhesions. Ischaemic heart disease, peripheral vascular disease and atrial fibrillation are all associated with mesenteric ischaemia.

Drugs and alcohol

These are an important part of a history and should be explored with the patient, family or a general practitioner.

EXAMINATION

General physical examination is necessary, particularly as patients may require surgery and an assessment of anaesthetic risk can be made. The state of hydration must be established as profound third space loss can occur and replacement requirements can be large.

Continued monitoring of temperature, pulse and blood pressure is important as often an exact diagnosis cannot be made, but signs of the patient's condition worsening may simply be a rising pulse or falling blood pressure.

Surgical emphysema in the neck is associated with a ruptured oesophagus and rapidly points to this diagnosis when detected.

Abdominal examination

Abdominal examination should begin with inspection of the position the patient adopts in the bed as there is a reluctance to move when there is peritonitis and a flexed right hip may suggest inflammation around the appendix. Peritoneal irritation (peritonism) is demonstrated by rebound tenderness and guarding. Then look for pulsation or masses, surgical scars and hernias.

Palpation should localise areas of maximal tenderness, area of guarding and the board-like rigidity of the abdominal wall following a perforated ulcer.

Abdominal auscultation is principally for the de-tection of bowel sounds which disappear with peritonitis and are tinkling when associated with small bowel obstruction. Bruits may be heard when there is mes-enteric ischaemia or aortic disease. Digital examination of the anorectal canal is mandatory.

Consideration should be given to abdominal pain that is caused by pathology outside the abdominal cavity and abdominal pathology that can cause pain outside the abdomen. Diaphragmatic irritation can present exclusively with shoulder tip pain – either right or left depending on which side the hemidiaphragm is irritated. Pleural irritation due to pulmonary infection or infarction can, on occasion, lead to a feeling of epigastric pain.

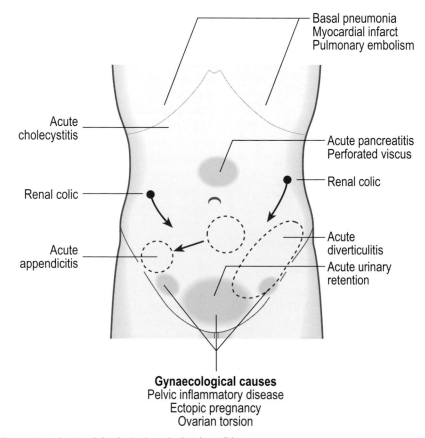

Basal pneumonia
Myocardial infarct
Pulmonary embolism

Acute cholecystitis

Acute pancreatitis
Perforated viscus

Renal colic

Renal colic

Acute diverticulitis

Acute appendicitis

Acute urinary retention

Gynaecological causes
Pelvic inflammatory disease
Ectopic pregnancy
Ovarian torsion

Fig. 1 **Sites of acute abdominal pain and related conditions.**

INVESTIGATION

Simple investigations such as full blood count and biochemistry are usually helpful in managing the patient but not in making a diagnosis. Useful diagnostic tests are a blood glucose and pH assessment in diabetic ketoacidosis, which may cause marked abdominal pain, and serum amylase count in acute pancreatitis.

An erect chest X-ray, including the diaphragm, is usually used to detect pneumonia and sub-diaphragmatic air in perforated hollow organs (Fig. 2). An erect abdominal X-ray may reveal fluid levels associated with intestinal obstruction or calcification in the wall of an aortic aneurysm or in the body of the pancreas in chronic pancreatitis.

History, examination and the above investigations should yield a diagnosis in the majority of patients or at least demonstrate the necessity or otherwise of laparotomy. This is a largely clinical decision and is usually essential in the presence of:

- acute appendicitis
- peritonitis (generalised or localised and severe)
- leaking abdominal aortic aneurysm
- ischaemic bowel
- intestinal obstruction (if it does not respond to simple measures).

Further investigations which may become necessary include abdominal ultrasound, CT and unprepared ('instant') enema. Laparoscopy is particularly useful in women of child-bearing age with lower abdominal pain.

MANAGEMENT

Regardless of the diagnosis patients should be promptly resuscitated with fluid or blood if appropriate. This may run in parallel with more definitive surgical treatment when this is required immediately as in a leaking aortic aneurysm, but usually should precede surgery.

Patients should be kept nil by mouth, and given sufficient analgesia for comfort (but not so much as to make clinical assessment impossible) and broad-spectrum, intravenous antibiotics when sepsis is suspected. Gram-negative sepsis and subsequent cardiovascular collapse can occur with startling rapidity and aggres-

sive management of fluid balance with central venous monitoring and replacement when necessary, and urinary output monitoring with prompt correction of oliguria, will help prevent the resultant downward spiral of hypotension, oliguria and renal failure.

Specific management of gastrointestinal causes of acute abdominal pain will be dealt with in other sections.

Diagnostic pitfalls which are not uncommon and can be avoided are:

- treating patients for renal colic when they have a leaking abdominal aortic aneurysm – which becomes apparent when the cardiovascular system collapses
- missing a femoral hernia as a cause of small bowel obstruction
- assuming a mechanical obstruction when there is colonic pseudo-obstruction
- performing a laparotomy when Münchausen's syndrome is the correct diagnosis.

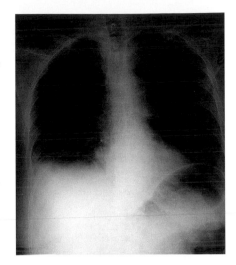

Fig. 2 **Sub-diaphragmatic gas following perforated hollow organ.**

Table 1 **Characteristic clinical features of enlarged organs**

Organ enlarged	Clinical features
Liver	Enlarges from RUQ, may be smooth/irregular, firm/hard. Left or caudate lobe may be palpable in epigastrium as a mass. Pulsatile in tricuspid regurgitation. Audible bruit in vascular tumours, tricuspid regurgitation, alcoholic hepatitis
Spleen	Enlarges from LUQ towards the right iliac fossa when very large. Dull to percussion. Has a palpable notch. Non-ballottable. Cannot get above it because of the ribs. Dullness to percussion over the lower ribs
Kidneys	Ballottable. Resonant if there is overlying bowel gas. Irregular in the presence of cysts or tumour
Bladder	Arises from the pelvis. Dull to percussion. Tender if acute outflow obstruction
Ovary	Arises from pelvis. Dull to percussion

The clinical approach

- Establish the characteristics of the pain – site, onset, severity, nature, progression, duration and ending, aggravating/relieving factors, radiation.
- Include all portions of the history including past medical and surgical, family and drug history.
- Systematically examine the abdomen and demonstrate evidence of peritonism.
- Think about pathology within the abdomen that causes symptoms elsewhere, and about pathology outside the abdomen that causes symptoms within.
- Formulate a differential diagnosis and direct investigations accordingly.
- A decision to perform a laparotomy is largely a clinical decision.

ACUTE PANCREATITIS

CLINICAL FEATURES

The condition is characterised by an acute inflammatory reaction in the pancreas which results in an abrupt onset of severe upper abdominal pain. There is acinar damage, with enzyme leak resulting in autodigestion and microcirculatory changes, an acute inflammatory infiltrate and fat necrosis. Activation of trypsinogen to trypsin is thought to be an important step as this appears to activate kinins and complement.

Severity ranges from mild, self-limiting attacks to severe episodes with multiple organ involvement and an overall mortality of 10–15%.

The diagnosis is made when there is acute onset of abdominal pain accompanied by at least a three-fold increase in the serum amylase or lipase level. However, normal amylase levels may be seen in acute pancreatitis caused by hyperlipidaemia, and elevated levels can be due to malignant conditions affecting the colon, lung and ovaries. 10% of chronic alcoholics have salivary derived hyperamylasaemia which may lead to diagnostic difficulties in alcoholics with abdominal pain. Serum lipase activity may be a slightly more sensitive test and levels may remain elevated for longer after an attack. Persistently elevated levels of amylase after an acute episode may indicate the development of a pancreatic pseudocyst.

Patients may have signs associated with an acute abdomen and there may be signs of cholangitis when due to biliary stones. There is frequently tachycardia and hypotension owing to hypovolaemia. Discoloration of the skin resulting from extravasation of pancreatic juice into the flanks (Grey Turner's sign) or around the umbilicus (Cullen's sign) may occur.

In addition to clinical suspicion and elevated serum amylase or lipase level, chest and abdominal X-rays should be performed to exclude other pathology such as intestinal obstruction or perforated viscus and to aid staging and diagnosis. The chest X-ray may show pleural effusions (Fig. 1), features of adult respiratory distress syndrome in severe cases or sub-diaphragmatic gas in perforated viscus. Abdominal X-ray may show a

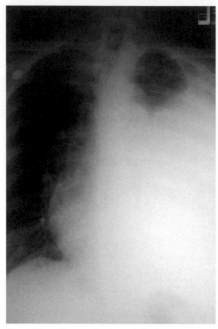

Fig. 1 **Chest X-ray with pleural effusion.**

local ileus around the pancreas (sentinel loop) or calcified gallstones which may be helpful but are non-specific.

Abdominal ultrasound is necessary to visualise a swollen or necrotic pancreas, but because of overlying bowel gas, the view is poor in up to 50% of cases. It is useful for detecting free peritoneal fluid and seeking evidence of gallstones as this is important for subsequent management decisions regarding ERCP.

CT scanning is not usually necessary for diagnosis but is useful when assessing more severe cases to detect the development of pancreatic necrosis or peripancreatic fluid.

Biliary stones and alcohol abuse account for 75% of cases of acute pancreatitis but there are many other causes (Table 1). Even with careful assessment, 20% of cases remain idiopathic.

Assessment of disease severity

It is recommended that patients are stratified for disease severity within 48 hours of admission. A number of scoring systems have been described which use clinical and biochemical parameters. The Glasgow scoring system with CRP is widely used for initial assessment (Table 2). CRP above 210 mg/l in the first 4 days or > 120 mg/l at the end of the first week signifies a severe attack.

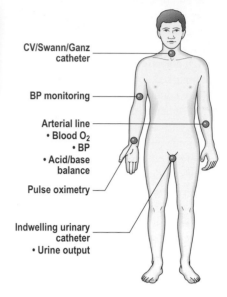

Fig. 2 **Monitoring of patient with acute pancreatitis.**

MANAGEMENT

Patients with mild attacks, around 80% of cases, are monitored routinely (pulse, blood pressure, temperature and urine output), and are treated with intravenous fluids and analgesia, and are kept nil by mouth (Fig. 2). This approach usually ensures a full recovery.

Those experiencing severe attacks need careful resuscitation to try to prevent early respiratory, cardiac or renal failure. In addition to the above measures the following should be used:

- central venous pressure measurement and fluid replacement
- urine output monitoring, and renal support if necessary
- nasogastric tube
- blood gas estimation and correction of hypoxia with O_2 or mechanical ventilation and monitoring of pH balance
- Swan–Ganz catheter placement in patients with circulatory failure.

Infected pancreatic necrosis is a severe complication which may require surgical lavage but there appear to be specific benefits to outcome if the antibiotic imipenem is used early in severe disease. Multiple organ failure may occur with impaired renal function because of hypovolaemia, hypoxia and ultimately the development of adult respiratory distress syndrome. Peptic ulcer disease and

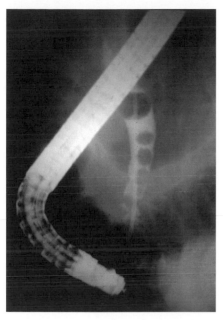

Fig. 3 **Bile duct stones trawled with a balloon.**

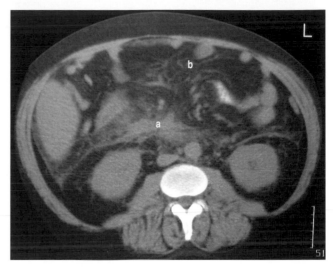

Fig. 4 **CT scan with acute pancreatitis (a) and widespread fat necrosis (b).**

gastritis can result in GI haemorrhage, and pleural effusions may develop, particularly left-sided exudates with a high amylase. Metabolic abnormalities are common with hypocalcaemia, hyperglycaemia and hypertrygyceridaemia. As prolonged recovery will be accompanied by malnourishment, intravenous feeding may be required.

If there is evidence of biliary stones or sepsis, or in acute severe pancreatitis biliary stones may be present, then ERCP should be performed early and the bile duct cleared of stones (Fig. 3).

Assessment of the pancreas for evidence of necrosis, abscess or pseudocyst development can be by ultrasound or CT (Fig. 4). Infected necrosis, if not responding to conservative measures, may need drainage either under radiological control or by laparotomy. Abscess formation may occur as a late complication and also needs drainage.

Pancreatic pseudocysts are pancreatic juice filled sacs which may be connected to the pancreatic duct. They may regress spontaneously or be complicated by infection or haemorrhage. Drainage can be performed percutaneously under ultrasound control or endoscopically if adjacent to the stomach by the placement of a stent from the pseudocyst cavity into the gastric lumen.

Following recovery, assessment of the bile duct should be performed if there is evidence of gallstones. If there is no evidence and the attack was mild then ERCP is probably not justified. Cholecystectomy should be performed if

gallstones were thought to be causative, in order to prevent further attacks, ideally within 4 weeks of the patient's recovery following mild attacks but later after severe episodes. If there is no identified aetiology and attacks are recurrent, ERCP should be performed to detect predisposing anatomical variations.

Table 1 **Causes of acute pancreatitis**

- Biliary stones
- Alcohol
- Hyperlipidaemia
- Hereditary pancreatitis (autosomal dominant)
- Hyperparathyroidism and hypercalcaemia
- Drugs
    azathioprine and 6-mercaptopurine
    sulphasalazine
    olsalazine
    antibiotics: metronidazole, tetracycline,
        nitrofurantoin
    valproic acid
    corticosteroids
    frusemide
- Anatomic abnormalities
    pancreas divisum (non-fusion of dorsal and
    ventral ducts)
    sphincter of Oddi dysfunction
- Trauma
- Iatrogenic
    post-ERCP
    postoperative
- Infections
    mumps, Coxsackie B, CMV
    TB, leptospirosis
- Scorpion venom

Strong advice regarding alcohol consumption should be given if necessary.

Special mention should be made of patients following ERCP. Pancreatitis affects less than 10% of procedures of which a small percentage are serious, but this complication accounts for a significant proportion of ERCP-related deaths. Careful assessment of the patient for abdominal pain, tachycardia and hypotension should be made in the hours following ERCP and if present, patients should be resuscitated with fluids, kept nil by mouth and started on intravenous imipenem. Post-ERCP pancreatitis in patients with sphincter of Oddi dysfunction is particularly common and patients must be counselled accordingly.

Table 2 **Prognostic factors for acute pancreatitis**

Criteria of severity within the first 24 hours

Age > 55
WBC > 15 × 10⁹/l
Blood glucose > 10 mmol/l
Urea > 16 mmol/l
paO_2 < 8 kPa
Serum calcium < 2.0 mmol/l
Serum albumin < 32 g/l
Serum lactate dehydrogenase > 600 u/l
Aspartate transaminase > 100 u/l

Acute pancreatitis

- Clinical suspicion and raised serum amylase level are usually enough to establish a diagnosis of acute pancreatitis but other conditions may lead to a rise in the amylase and not all cases of acute pancreatitis are accompanied by hyperamylasaemia.
- Careful clinical and biochemical assessment of patients with acute pancreatitis is mandatory early in its presentation.
- 80% of cases are mild and patients make an uneventful recovery. 10–15% experience severe attacks and may die from acute pancreatitis.
- Careful ITU monitoring is required for patients with severe pancreatitis.
- ERCP is required for patients with evidence of gallstone pancreatitis.
- CT imaging is useful to detect complications such as necrosis, abscess formation or pseudocyst development.

ACUTE APPENDICITIS / DIVERTICULAR DISEASE

ACUTE APPENDICITIS

Appendicitis is more commonly seen in Western countries and affects men more than women. It is uncommon in the very young (under 2 years) and the elderly. There are two main causes:

- **Non-obstructive acute appendicitis** occurs as a result of inflammation within the mucous membrane lining the appendix.

- **Obstructive appendicitis** (about 80%) occurs due to obstruction of the lumen most commonly by a faecolith.

  In appendicitis, the appendix becomes distended with bacteria and the products of inflammation. This tends to develop more rapidly when the lumen is obstructed. Often the appendix distal to the point of obstruction will become gangrenous and if untreated will perforate.

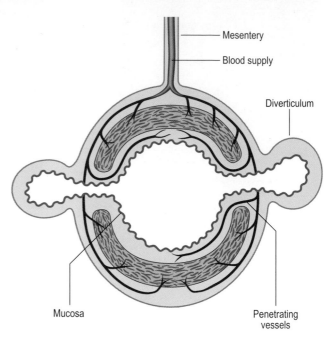

Fig. 1 **Anatomy of diverticulae in the colon.**

CLINICAL FEATURES

As the appendix becomes distended, the initial presentation is with peri-umbilical pain. This is pain which is referred to the site of embryonic origin. As inflammation progresses, the appendix starts to irritate the overlying parietal peritoneum and pain develops in the right iliac fossa (RIF). Later on this may be associated with localised guarding and rebound tenderness.

There may also be an associated systemic upset with anorexia, nausea, vomiting and occasionally diarrhoea.

Outcome from appendicitis will often depend upon the speed at which inflammation and suppuration develop. When the lumen of the appendix is not obstructed appendicitis may resolve without treatment. Failing this, non-obstructive appendicitis may proceed relatively slowly allowing the appendix to become walled off by omentum, caecum and small bowel. Such patients may present with a tender palpable mass in the RIF (appendix mass) which may eventually develop into an abscess (Table 1). If the appendicitis proceeds more rapidly, there may not be sufficient time for surrounding organs to wall off the appendix. If the appendix perforates then peritonitis develops.

DIFFERENTIAL DIAGNOSIS

This is primarily from Crohn's ileitis, pyelonephritis, perforated peptic ulcer, acute cholecystitis, intestinal obstruction (particularly if due to caecal carcinoma) and gastroenteritis. In children, mesenteric lymphadenitis associated with an upper respiratory tract infection should be considered. In women, pelvic inflammatory disease, torsion of an ovarian cyst and ectopic pregnancy need to be excluded.

EXAMINATION

The patient may be non-specifically unwell with a temperature and vague abdominal pain. In more advanced cases there may be features of peritonism – rebound tenderness in which pressure in the left iliac fossa can induce pain in the right iliac fossa (Rovsing's sign) and following release of the pressure pain is produced in the right (Blumberg's sign). The patient may adopt a position with the right hip slightly flexed if the appendix is resting on and irritating the right psoas muscle. Coughing and sudden movement can generate localised pain. If the appendix is retrocaecal the tenderness may be in the lateral part of the lumbar region, and a subhepatic appendix can produce pain and tenderness in the right upper quadrant.

Table 1 **Differential diagnosis of a mass in the right iliac fossa**

Appendix mass
Caecal carcinoma
Caecum distended with faeces
Crohn's disease of the terminal ileum
Ileocaecal tuberculosis
Psoas abscess
Pelvic kidney
Ovarian mass
Aneurysm of the common or external iliac artery
Retroperitoneal tumour
Distended gallbladder

Rectal examination may produce pain in the pelvis when pressure with the examining finger is directed towards the right iliac fossa. Extension of the right hip may produce pain, and children may limp due to this discomfort.

INVESTIGATION

Investigation may be largely unnecessary in the straightforward case. In less clear cases some tests may be useful to exclude other diagnoses. There is usually a leucocytosis. Pregnancy testing and urine testing for infection may be helpful. Ultrasound of the right iliac fossa is the first diagnostic test for patients with a mass in the right iliac fossa.

TREATMENT

Following rehydration with intravenous fluids, the administration of prophylactic antibiotics (metronidazole) and possibly

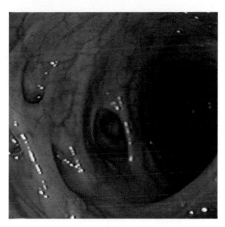

Fig. 2 **Sigmoidoscopy showing diverticulae.**

anti-DVT prophylaxis (low molecular weight heparin), the patient is taken to theatre. The appendix is removed and any localised abscess drained. If there is evidence of peritonitis then the abdomen is thoroughly lavaged.

Postoperatively, the patient receives intravenous fluids until drinking. In addition, if the appendix is gangrenous or perforated then they should also receive intravenous antibiotics of a cephalosporin and metronidazole.

DIVERTICULAR DISEASE

The wall of the colon has a complete circular muscle coat and also a longitudinal coat arranged in strips known as *taenia coli*. The circular muscle coat is pierced by blood vessels. Diverticulae are acquired herniations of the colonic mucosa through the circular muscle coat at the site where blood vessels enter (Fig. 1). Colonic diverticulae are seen predominantly in Western countries and are thought to reflect a diet low in fibre. The stool in such patients tends to be of low volume and firm or hard, resulting in a raised intraluminal pressure and muscular incoordination which leads to the development of colonic diverticulae.

CLINICAL PICTURE

This varies depending upon the presence or absence of complications.

- The majority of patients have few symptoms. They may have a history of an erratic bowel habit and occasional discomfort in the left iliac fossa (LIF).
- Inflammation within one or more diverticulae leads to the diverticulitis. Patients have more persistent

abdominal pain, usually in the left iliac fossa. Bowel habit will be variable. They may have evidence of a systemic upset with malaise, fever and a leucocytosis.

- If the diverticulum perforates it may develop a pericolic abscess or may lead to generalised peritonitis. The patient will have increasing abdominal pain with either a localised tender mass (usually in the LIF) or evidence of peritonitis. The systemic upset will be more pronounced.
- The inflamed diverticulum may become walled off by other organs with the development of a fistula into the bladder (vesicocolic), uterus (uterocolic) or small bowel (enterocolic). Patients with a vesicocolic fistula may notice bubbles of air in the urine (pneumaturia).
- Because diverticulae develop where the bowel wall is pierced by blood vessels, an inflamed diverticulum may erode through a vessel wall resulting in profuse colonic haemorrhage.

DIAGNOSIS

Radiology

In the acute case, endoscopy and contrast radiology should be avoided because of the risk of perforating an acutely inflamed bowel. CT scanning has a high diagnostic yield and ultrasound may be of value if a pericolic abscess is suspected. Usually the diagnosis is made by double contrast barium enema, following settling of the acute attack. This visualises the diverticulae and helps to

exclude other causes such as malignancy.

Endoscopy

Whilst diverticulae are easily seen at sigmoidoscopy the main use is in differentiating benign from malignant strictures (Fig. 2).

MANAGEMENT

Conservative

The majority of patients with diverticular disease have no or minor symptoms and can be managed with a high fibre diet and bulk laxatives. If symptoms suggest acute diverticulitis then a broad-spectrum antibiotic should be added. For the patient who has had an uncomplicated recovery a conservative approach should be adopted once the diagnosis has been confirmed.

Surgical

For patients who have repeated episodes of acute diverticulitis the ideal approach is a one-stage resection. As the sigmoid is the area most commonly affected the procedure is usually a sigmoid colectomy.

A pericolic abscess can usually be drained under ultrasound or CT guidance and an elective resection performed at a later date. If radiological drainage is not possible then the abscess will need to be drained at operation, during which the affected segment of bowel should also be removed. In this situation, primary re-anastomosis is more hazardous and it is safer to bring out the proximal end as a colostomy. The distal end is closed (Hartmann's procedure). Re-anastomosis can be performed at a later date once the sepsis has resolved.

Fistulae are treated by resection of the diseased bowel and closure of the fistula.

Acute appendicitis/diverticular disease

- Acute appendicitis is a common condition and can be considered in all but the very young and the very old.
- The diagnosis is easy when the clinical signs are typical but can be very difficult when atypical.
- Retrocaecal appendix and subhepatic appendix can lead to diagnostic confusion.
- Complications of pregnancy and urinary tract infection should be excluded.
- Diverticulae become common with age and are usually asymptomatic.
- Diverticulae can perforate, lead to obstruction, cause fistulae and haemorrhage.

THE CLINICAL APPROACH

DEFINITION OF DIARRHOEA

Although perhaps not the most glamorous of topics in gastroenterology, diarrhoea is undoubtedly important because an estimated 10% of general practitioner consultations are for diarrhoeal illnesses and, worldwide, it may be the second most common cause of death – particularly amongst children in developing countries.

Chronic diarrhoea is defined as lasting longer than 4 weeks, and acute diarrhoea as lasting less than this. Patients tend to think of diarrhoea as passing stools with a more fluid consistency without particular change in frequency, whereas medical interest should be in both, and a definition should include an increase in frequency above three times a day with decreased consistency and, traditionally, an increased stool weight above 250 g per day.

PHYSIOLOGY OF STOOL FLUID BALANCE

Normally, 2 litres (or more) of water are ingested per day, which, added to the 7 litres of secretions from salivery glands, stomach, bile and pancreas, totals 9 litres per day passing into the small intestine. 7.5 litres are absorbed by the small intestine, leaving just over 1 litre to be absorbed by the colon. This represents approximately 20% of total body water and so it can be readily seen that minor imbalances in this system can rapidly lead to profound dehydration.

Sodium movement across the luminal border of the small intestine controls water movement by osmosis. Na^+ absorption from the lumen facilitates glucose absorption, whilst K^+ diffuses back into the lumen. This explains why diarrhoea can lead to hypokalaemia and why sodium and glucose replacement is effective in treating hypovolaemia following diarrhoea (Table 1).

PATHOPHYSIOLOGICAL MECHANISMS OF DIARRHOEA

It is useful to classify diarrhoea into four groups which have different mechanisms of production and causes (Table 2).

Osmotic diarrhoea

Non-absorbed solutes which are osmoti-
cally active will prevent water absorption from the intestinal lumen. These are usually poorly digested carbohydrates or lipids. This type of diarrhoea will stop during fasting or when the solute is no longer ingested. To confirm an osmotic diarrhoea, the osmotic gap between actual and usual stool osmolarity is calculated:

Stool osmolarity = $2(\text{stool } Na^+ + K^+) - 300$ (normal stool osmolarity).

An osmotic gap greater than 100 suggests an osmotic diarrhoea.

Secretory diarrhoea

Failure of adequate intestinal absorption or increased secretion results in a secretory diarrhoea. Failure of adequate absorption is most common and can be as a result of mucosal disease or resection, whilst active secretion can be stimulated by bacterial toxins, stimulant laxatives or hormones. This type of diarrhoea does not stop during fasting and does not demonstrate a marked osmotic gap.

Inflammatory/exudative diarrhoea

Gut inflammation disrupts the integrity of the mucosa resulting in fluid loss into the lumen. There may also be a secretory element because inflammatory mediators may also stimulate secretion.

Dysmotility diarrhoea

Abnormal gut motility may also cause diarrhoea because decreased transit times allow insufficient time for adequate fluid absorption. This alone may cause diarrhoea but is unlikely to cause increased stool weights; however, dysmotility often coexists with other mechanisms for diarrhoea production.

HISTORY

Unless the history is approached in a systematic way, the clinician will become bewildered by patients with diarrhoea. It is more important to establish whether the diarrhoea is acute or chronic and fatty, watery or bloody, because this approach will allow appropriate investigation .

Acute diarrhoea

An abrupt onset associated with vomiting, systemic upset and clustering with other
individuals, points to an infective cause for the diarrhoea. A self-limiting illness lasting a few days with a watery diarrhoea suggests either a viral cause or *E. coli*. Bloody diarrhoea may be caused by infection with *Salmonella*, *Shigella* or *Campylobacter*.

Chronic diarrhoea

Fatty stools

A history of passing poorly formed pale stools which have a particularly offensive aroma, are difficult to flush from the toilet and occasionally contain fat globules suggests a fatty stool or steatorrhoea. Steatorrhoea implies malabsorption or maldigestion and the major causes of these are gluten-sensitive enteropathy (coeliac disease/sprue), which results in malabsorption, and chronic exocrine pancreatic insufficiency, which results in maldigestion. Other less frequent causes include *Giardia* infestation, Whipple's disease, α-chain disease and scleroderma.

Watery stools

If the stool is watery and of high volume (>1 l) which does not fall on fasting, a secretory cause is suggested. Lower volumes which do abate on fasting imply an osmotic process. Normal volumes with a small increase in frequency and decrease in consistency suggest a dysmotility cause.

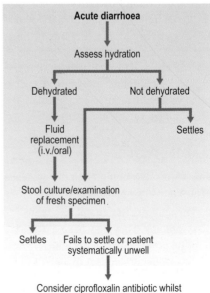

Fig. 1 **Investigation algorithm for acute diarrhoea.**

Bloody diarrhoea/blood in the stools

When patients describe passage of blood, it is important to determine whether or not there has been a change in the stools or simply the passage of blood with an otherwise normal stool. Blood and diarrhoea suggest a colonic cause for the symptoms, such as inflammation, whereas normal stools with blood should prompt a search for a local cause such as haemorrhoids or rectal disease.

Other important symptoms should be sought, such as soiling, urgency, a sensation of incomplete evacuation, pain or abdominal cramps and bloating. There are a number of sinister symptoms that should always be sought; these include nocturnal diarrhoea, weight loss, bleeding and the presence of associated rashes and arthropathy.

Having established the nature of the diarrhoea, careful inquiry is essential, into:

- **medication** – both prescribed and self-administered
- **diet** – including alcohol and coffee
- **previous surgery** and obstetric history
- **pre-existing illnesses** such as diabetes or scleroderma
- **family history**.

Sexual proclivity and practice should be established.

EXAMINATION

When examining a patient with an acute diarrhoeal illness, first establish the state of fluid balance because dehydration can be profound. Tachycardia, hypotension or a postural drop, dry mucous membranes and increased skin turgor point to this.

A more general examination should look for skin rashes and flushing, evidence of a synovitis, abdominal tenderness, masses and bruits. Rectal examination, in addition to allowing the detection of tumours, will also demonstrate the state of stool. Rigid sigmoidoscopy on an unprepared bowel also allows stool visualisation and examination and biopsy of rectal mucosa.

Table 1 **Fluid and electrolyte replacement (Electrolade)**

236 mg sodium chloride
300 mg potassium chloride
500 mg sodium bicarbonate
4 g glucose
Reconstitute in 200 ml water. Adults should consume 1–2 sachets after each loose stool (maximum 16 in 24 hours) and children over 2 years, 1 sachet after each loose stool (maximum 12 in 24 hours)

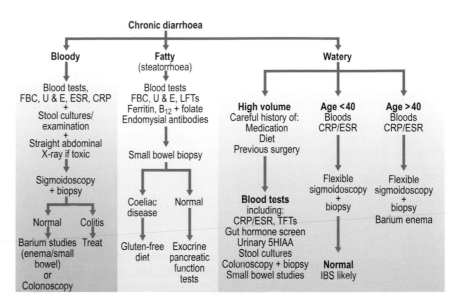

Fig. 2 **Investigation algorithm for chronic diarrhoea.**

INVESTIGATIONS

In an **acute diarrhoea**, full blood count and white cell differential will detect anaemia and demonstrate a lymphocytosis, which suggests a viral cause, and neutrophilia, which suggests an inflammatory cause – however, a neutropenia can occur with salmonellosis. Biochemistry helps assess hydration. Inflammatory markers – ESR and CRP – may be elevated when there is systemic infection, and blood cultures should be performed in the presence of a pyrexia. A straight abdominal X-ray is performed in the toxic patient to detect megacolon, which may complicate acute severe ulcerative colitis and also pseudomembranous colitis. Stool culture is routinely taken but may be unhelpful because many acute diarrhoeas are caused by viruses that are not routinely detected in stool specimens. Fresh stool samples are required for microscopic examination for amoebae. The investigation of patients with **chronic diarrhoea** is initially similar to that for acute diarrhoea.

Table 2 **Classification and causes of diarrhoea**

Type	Causes
Osmotic diarrhoea	Carbohydrate malabsorption (lactase deficiency)
	Sodium- or anion-containing laxatives or those containing magnesium
	Excessive intake of poorly absorbed carbohydrates (lactulose, sorbitol, fructose)
	Intestinal mucosal disease (coeliac disease or tropical sprue)
Secretory diarrhoea	Bacterial infections with enterotoxins (cholera, enterotoxigenic *E. coli*)
	Stimulant laxatives (bisacodyl, cascara, docusate, senna)
	Hormones (carcinoid, VIPoma, gastrinoma)
	Microscopic colitis (collagenous, lymphocytic)
	Bile acid malabsorption (terminal ileal resection, Crohn's disease)
	Villous adenoma of the rectum
Inflammatory diarrhoea	Infections without enterotoxins (viruses, bacteria, parasites)
	Inflammatory bowel disease (Ulcerative colitis, Crohn's, Behçet's)
	Ischaemia
Dysmotility diarrhoea	Irritable bowel syndrome
	Endocrine disease (hyperthyroidism, phaeochromocytoma)
	Autonomic neuropathy (diabetes)

The clinical approach

- Establish from the history whether the presentation of diarrhoea is acute or chronic and whether the stools are bloody, watery or fatty.
- Establish what surgery has been performed previously — particularly previous intestinal resections.
- As always, a thorough drug history is required.
- If the patient is young and there are no sinister features in the history, irritable bowel syndrome is the most likely diagnosis.
- Rectal bleeding, weight loss and a change in bowel habit in the older age group always require investigation — particularly to exclude neoplasia.

COELIAC DISEASE (COELIAC SPRUE)

Coeliac disease, coeliac sprue (in the USA) or gluten-sensitive enteropathy is a condition characterised by disorders of the small intestine that result from an intolerance to dietary gluten in susceptible individuals.

Coeliac disease was originally thought to present in childhood with the classic symptoms of failure to thrive, steatorrhoea, and occasionally osteomalacia, all beginning when children were being weaned from milk to solids. It is now clear that the condition can either be unrecognised in adults or remain latent until triggered by some environmental event, well into late adult life, and now occasionally the diagnosis is made in patients of 70 or 80 who have presented with an iron deficiency anaemia.

PREVALENCE

The quoted prevalence of the condition has wide geographic variation with levels of 1 : 1200 in the UK up to 1 : 300 in western Ireland. However, it is now becoming clear that when aggressive screening programmes are undertaken, prevalence levels rise to 1 : 250 in the USA and even 1 : 152 in Ireland. This has led to the description of a coeliac iceberg (Fig. 1) with the majority of patients either having unrecognised or latent coeliac disease.

AETIOLOGY

The condition is caused by an alcohol-soluble component (gliadin) found in the gluten fraction of wheat. Similarly, active elements in rye, barley and oats can induce the condition and need to be avoided in the diet of sufferers (Table 1).

There is a genetic predisposition to the condition; monozygotic twins have almost 100% concordance and first-degree relatives of affected individuals have a 10–20% risk of developing the condition. It is now also apparent that coeliac disease

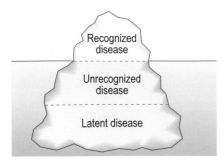

Fig. 1 **The coeliac iceberg.**

is an HLA-associated condition, particularly with HLA-DQ2, -DQ8 and -DQ4. It is not clear why individuals with these associations should develop clinical coeliac disease, particularly as a quarter of the normal population express HLA-DQ2.

PATHOLOGY

The histological changes seen vary widely in severity and extent. There is an increase in intraepithelial lymphocytes, predominantly T cells, villous atrophy and crypt hyperplasia (Fig. 2). However, as more subtle presentations of the condition are recognised, an increase in intraepithelial lymphocytes may be the only change seen. Small bowel biopsies were originally collected using a Crosby capsule, which was passed into the jejunum under X-ray screening. Biopsies are now more usually obtained at the time of upper GI endoscopy because distal duodenal biopsies invariably demonstrate abnormalities seen more distally in the small bowel.

SEROLOGY

The original serological tests were with IgG and IgA antibodies to gliadin (AGA). IgG AGA is not particularly sensitive and may be positive in other GI conditions and also in some healthy individuals. IgA AGA is more sensitive and specific but both tests have been superseded by anti-endomysial antibodies (AEA). IgA AEA is most useful but has the drawback that up to 10% of patients with coeliac disease have a selective IgA deficiency which renders the test useless; IgG AEA should be assayed in these patients.

CLINICAL FEATURES

In children, the presentation is usually with anorexia, abdominal distension, diarrhoea and failure to gain weight. Adult patients may present with diarrhoea and weight loss, but many just have anaemia or metabolic bone disease. Some are now being picked up following screening in patient groups whose condition is associated with a high incidence of coeliac disease, such as those with insulin-dependent diabetes or thyroid disease (Table 2).

DIAGNOSIS

The diagnosis enters the differential in many circumstances, and screening for coeliac disease has been made easier with serological testing. In an individual with a positive serology test, small bowel biopsies should be undertaken on a normal diet and ideally repeated after 3–6 months on a gluten-free diet (GFD). Demonstration of improvement in the biopsy appearance confirms the diagnosis.

COMPLICATIONS

Malignancy

A number of complications of coeliac disease may occur, particularly intestinal malignancy and lymphoma, and it is not uncommon for coeliac disease to be recognised after the diagnosis of intestinal lymphoma has been made. These lymphomas are usually of T cell origin, which corresponds with the increase in intraepithelial T lymphocytes that occurs in the small bowel of patients with coeliac disease. The occurrence of these malignancies probably explains the doubling of the mortality of patients with coeliac disease compared to the general population. There appears to be a reduction in the risk with close adherence to a GFD, which is another reason for patients to adhere closely to the diet.

Ulcerative jejunitis

Ulcerative jejunitis is a condition where there is mucosal ulceration and, potentially, haemorrhage, scarring and stricturing which may be a complication, or a variant, of coeliac disease. Treatment may require surgical resection in addition to a GFD.

Metabolic bone disease

Metabolic bone disease has long been recognised to be associated with coeliac disease but was thought to be predominantly osteomalacia. It is now clear that osteoporosis is also frequently associated and may occur in up to a quarter of patients with coeliac disease. This should be detected by X-ray absorptiometry to assess bone density and treated with either hormone replacement therapy if appropriate, or agents such as bisphosphonates.

Dermatitis herpetiformis (DH)

Although less than 10% of patients with coeliac disease have DH, virtually all

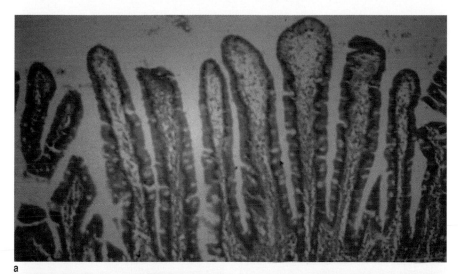

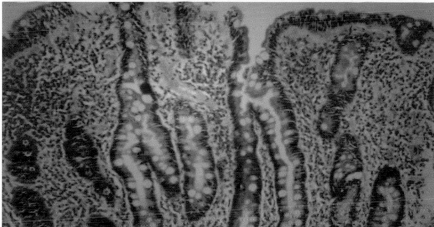

Fig. 2 Histological changes in coeliac disease. (a) normal villous architecture with long villi; (b) blunted villi of coeliac disease.

patients with DH have evidence of enteropathy. The clinical features are of an intensely itchy rash, particularly affecting the elbows and knees, with small vesicles that are denuded because of scratching. There is a characteristic deposition of IgA in the dermis, which is demonstrated at skin biopsy. There are similar HLA associations to those of coeliac disease. Treatment requires a GFD and may require dapsone, particularly in the early stages.

Lactase deficiency

An intolerance of lactose as a result of lactase deficiency is more common in coeliac disease patients than in the normal population and may complicate treatment of the condition. If suspected, a lactose hydrogen breath test can be undertaken or dairy products can simply be excluded from the diet for a trial period.

Splenic atrophy

This appears to be a relatively common complication of coeliac disease which predisposes patients to serious bacterial infection. Evidence for splenic atrophy is in the blood film, with the demonstration of Howell–Jolly bodies. Patients with hyposplenism should be advised to receive pneumococcal vaccination.

MANAGEMENT

The treatment of coeliac disease requires exclusion of wheat, rye, and probably oats from the diet. These either may be avoided completely or can be substituted with products made from maize or rice. Patients usually respond promptly with an improvement in their symptoms, but the histological changes in the small intestine take much longer to recover. The most common reason for patients to relapse is deliberate or inadvertent dietary lapse. This can usually be rectified by taking a close history and referral to a dietition. There is a small group of patients that do not respond to a GFD alone and may require treatment with corticosteroids. A concern in these patients is that an enteropathy-associated lymphoma is being missed.

At diagnosis, there may be deficiencies of iron, folic acid or vitamins and these should be supplemented initially but then can usually be stopped. Calcium and vitamin D may encourage improvement in osteoporosis, which frequently persists despite a GFD, and may be given long term.

Patients may, however, develop complications of coeliac disease that may present in a similar way to the underlying condition with diarrhoea and weight loss. This presents particular difficulty when a lymphoma develops because this can be a difficult diagnosis to either confirm or exclude.

It is appropriate to intermittently follow up these patients to encourage GFD adherence, keep a check on the patients' weight, monitor blood parameters and recognise complications that may develop.

Table 1 Acceptability of foodstuffs in coeliac disease

To be avoided	Acceptable
Wheat	Rice
Rye	Maize (corn)
Barley	Soya
Oats	Buckwheat
	Tapioca

Table 2 Conditions associated with coeliac disease

- Insulin-dependent diabetes mellitus
- Dermatitis herpetiformis
- Down's syndrome
- Epilepsy (particularly in the presence of cerebral calcification)
- IgA deficiency
- Autoimmune thyroid disease
- Atopic dermatitis
- Recurrent oral aphthous ulceration
- Primary biliary cirrhosis
- Sjögren's syndrome
- Sarcoidosis

Coeliac disease

- Coeliac disease is a condition that affects not only children, but also adults.
- It should be considered in patients with iron deficiency anaemia, diarrhoea and weight loss, as well as those with more characteristic features such as steatorrhoea.
- IgA anti-endomysial antibodies may be negative in patients with IgA deficiency, but it is otherwise a good screening test for coeliac disease.
- Coeliac disease is associated with conditions such as insulin-dependent diabetes, osteoporosis and thyroid disease.

ULCERATIVE COLITIS I

DEFINITION

Ulcerative colitis (UC) is a chronic inflammatory condition of unknown aetiology that affects the colon for a variable extent proximally from the rectum. Other systems such as eyes, skin and joints may be affected. The onset is usually gradual over a number of weeks with the major symptom being bloody diarrhoea.

EPIDEMIOLOGY

The peak age of presentation is in the 20–40 year range with a secondary peak in late middle age, although the condition may present at any age. The incidence ranges from 3–15 : 100 000.

It is probable that there is a genetic component to the development of ulcerative colitis. Certain groups such as Caucasians generally and Jewish populations specifically, seem more prone to developing the condition. Siblings and family members of those affected also have higher risks of developing the condition with approximately a 1% lifetime risk, whilst offspring of ulcerative colitis sufferers have about a 10% risk of developing the condition.

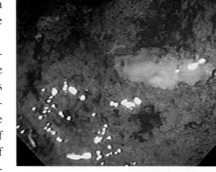

Fig. 1 **Inflamed rectal mucosa of UC.**

As yet, no consistent genetic abnormality has been identified, although many candidate genes have been studied. HLA associations have been made, particularly with HLA-DR2, but this has not been reliably reproduced.

The aetiology remains unknown, but various hypotheses have been made including abnormal colonic flora, abnormal colonic epithelium and an abnormal host immune response to the colonic flora. Environmental factors also play a part as it is clear that non-smokers are more prone to developing UC than smokers and those who have been heavy smokers are at particular risk of developing UC, especially within 2 years of stopping smoking.

NATURAL HISTORY

Presentation

The symptoms are of increased stool frequency, de-creased stool consistency, blood in the stool, tenesmus and mild abdominal pain.

Up to a third of patients at presentation have their entire colon affected, and it is usually this group that suffer the most severe symptoms and have the highest risk of going on to require surgery. The majority of patients have disease affecting just the rectum and sigmoid and have mild to moderate disease at presentation.

There is about a 10% risk of requiring colectomy in the first year after presentation, falling to 4% in the second year and falling further beyond that to 1% annually. After 10 years of disease, the chance of requiring surgery because of ongoing disease, not controlled by medical therapy, is low.

There is a slight-ly increased mortality in the first few years following presentation, largely owing to uncontrolled disease and surgery at the time of presentation, but survival then re-turns to normal values.

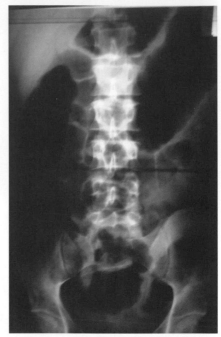

Fig. 2 **Megacolon visible on a straight abdominal X-ray.**

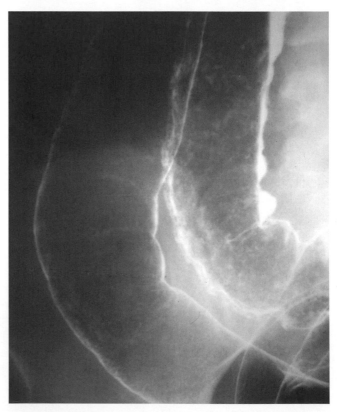

Fig. 3 **Barium enema showing the irregular mucosa of ulcerative colitis.**

Clinical course

In the majority of cases, the extent of involved colon remains static throughout the duration of the illness. However, about 10% of patients with distal disease have proximal extension to affect more of the colon.

10% have a single episode of colitis. The rest can have a

chronic intermittent course to their disease (the majority), a chronic continuous course (5–10%), or surgery (15–25%), and a very low percentage die because of their illness.

In a patient with active disease, there is a 70–80% chance of another flare-up within the next 12 months. If there has been a full year of remission, there is only a 20% chance of a flare-up in the next year. Activity of the disease appears to fall with increasing time.

DIFFERENTIAL DIAGNOSIS

In patients who present with bloody diarrhoea, the differential diagnosis is between an acute infective colitis, another type of chronic inflammatory bowel disease such as Crohn's disease or Behçet's disease, colorectal cancer and diverticular disease. Acute ischaemic colitis usually presents in the older age group with severe abdominal pain, associated with bloody diarrhoea.

Infective causes usually have a fairly abrupt onset, often associated with fever. All new presentations require stool cultures and if there is an antibiotic history then toxin assays should be performed for *Clostridium difficile*. Fresh stool samples are necessary to culture *Entamoeba histolytica* for diagnosis of amoebic dysentery in individuals who have travelled to the Far East, Africa and Central America.

Sigmoidoscopy and rectal biopsy can also help distinguish infective from chronic inflammatory causes, with histological features of chronicity present in ulcerative colitis.

Differentiation from a Crohn's colitis can be more difficult. Small bowel involvement, perianal disease, or characteristic histology helps differentiate between these two conditions. However, a small proportion of cases defy characterisation and, fortunately, as treatments are initially similar, this does not usually significantly affect medical management, but is significant if surgery is contemplated.

INVESTIGATIONS

Initial investigation should include full blood count, measurement of ESR and CRP, biochemistry and liver function tests. Stool culture with sigmoidoscopy and rectal biopsy are also required. In more severe cases with associated pyrexia, tachycardia and systemic upset, it is necessary to exclude dilatation of the colon, and straight abdominal X-ray is required.

Raised white cell count, platelet count, ESR or CRP levels point to severe or extensive disease. A non-specific rise in liver function tests may also occur with severe attacks and does not necessarily imply coexistent liver disease.

Sigmoidoscopy

Experience is necessary to first recognise normal rectal mucosa and then differentiate this from inflamed mucosa. With mild inflammation, the surface has a granular appearance as if sand has been sprinkled on to the moist surface. With more severe inflammation, the mucosa becomes friable with contact bleeding and in the most severe cases there is bleeding and ulceration (Fig. 1).

Histology

The histological features include an inflammatory infiltrate of neutro-phils, lymphocytes, plasma cells and macrophages, which is usually confined to the mucosa. Neutro-phils invade crypts causing 'cryptitis' and crypt abscesses. This inflammation results in mucus release from goblet cells with an appearance of goblet cell depletion. With chronic inflammation the architecture of the crypts is distorted, becoming branched, shortened and atrophied. These changes may persist even when the disease is in remission.

Radiology

At presentation, straight abdominal X-ray is performed to exclude dilatation of the colon which requires urgent attention as colonic perforation may be imminent. It is defined as dilatation of the colon of greater than 5.5 cm and may be associated with an irregular appearance of the mucosa, which is due to the presence of areas of relatively spared mucosa, termed 'mucosal islands' surrounded by deep ulceration (Fig. 2). Inflamed colon does not usually contain faeces and it has been suggested that faeces in the right colon implies more distal disease; this appears not to be the case as the plain radiograph underestimates disease extent.

Double-contrast barium enema should not be performed at presentation as this may cause colonic perforation. If necessary, an 'instant' enema (with an unprepared bowel) can help determine disease extent (Fig. 3). More elegantly, and without risk, white cell scanning outlines the inflamed colon more precisely (Fig. 4).

When the disease is in remission, barium enema may be performed to help determine disease extent, but with the widespread availability of colonoscopy, barium enema has largely been superseded.

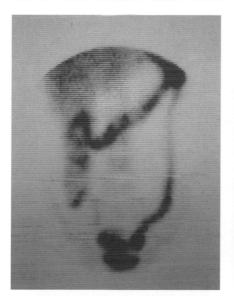

Fig. 4 **White cell scan showing increased activity throughout the colon in a patient with active UC.**

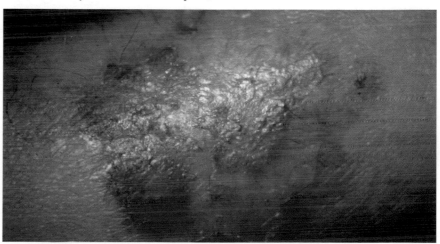

Fig. 5 **Pyderma gangrenosum seen in UC.**

ULCERATIVE COLITIS II

ASSOCIATED CONDITIONS

Skin

Pyoderma gangrenosum affects 1–2% of patients. It occurs on the trunk or limbs and may or may not reflect disease activity (Fig. 5, p. 47). Lesions are pustular and can break down with large areas of necrosis. **Erythema nodosum** appears as multiple tender nodules, looking like bruises usually on the shins. They occur in 2–4% of patients and may either occur with UC per se or complicate treatment with sulphasalazine (owing to the sulphapyridine group).

Liver

Persistent elevation of liver enzymes, particularly alkaline phosphatase and γ-glutamyl transferase (GGT) is characteristic of primary sclerosing cholangitis (PSC). This occurs in 2–10% of patients with UC and is characterised by strictures of the biliary tree. These may occur as pronounced strictures in the common bile duct or there may be multiple areas of narrowing, producing a beaded appearance, in intrahepatic bile ducts.

Symptoms may include itching or episodic jaundice, but often the diagnosis is made during the asymptomatic phase by detecting persistently abnormal liver function tests. Progression of the condition is unpredictable and does not reflect disease activity in the bowel. Diagnosis is usually best made at ERCP and there are characteristic histological changes, but owing to the patchy nature of the condition these may be missed at liver biopsy (see p. 93).

Treatment includes ursodeoxycholic acid, which leads to an improvement in LFTs and possibly slows the progression of the disease. Isolated troublesome strictures in the common bile duct can be treated endoscopically with balloon dilatation.

Cholangiocarcinoma is an important complication affecting up to 40% of patients with end-stage PSC. The diagnosis is suggested by a sudden increase in serum bilirubin level associated with weight loss and general deterioration in a patient with PSC. Confirming the diagnosis can be difficult because malignant strictures appear identical to benign. Brushings and biopsy at ERCP may help. The complication is usually fatal but early surgery offers a chance of cure.

Joints

Peripheral joints are quite frequently affected with arthralgia, particularly during disease exacerbations. Non-steroidal anti-inflammatory drugs should be avoided as these have been implicated in contributing to inflammatory bowel disease, and simple analgesics should be used. Sulphasalazine is probably the drug of choice for treatment of the colitis, if it can be tolerated, as it may specifically help the arthralgia. Sacroiliitis and ankylosing spondylitis are more important complications and affect 3–5% of patients with ulcerative colitis. They are strongly associated with HLA-B27. The condition runs a course separate to the colitis.

Eyes

Only 1–2% of patients develop eye problems. These include uveitis, which causes eye pain, photophobia and blurred vision and requires urgent ophthalmic attention, and episcleritis, which is less severe and responds to topical steroids.

Colorectal cancer

There is an increased risk of developing colorectal cancer, which appears to be related to disease extent and duration. The risk rises after approximately 10 years' duration of UC and particularly in patients with a pancolitis. Surveillance is usually reserved for this group of individuals, but demonstrating improved survival with surveillance has been difficult. Dysplastic changes in the colonic mucosa are sought and then monitored and the decision for colectomy is considered at this time. Maintenance treatment with ASA compounds (aminosalicylates) appears to reduce the risk of development of colorectal cancer.

Osteoporosis

This is an increasingly recognised complication, as a result of either the condition itself, or the use of corticosteroids. The availability of screening with X-ray absorptiometry and effective treatment now mean that the condition should be sought and treated.

TREATMENTS

Assessment of severity

At the time of the first presentation, assessment of extent is usually not possible (see 'Investigations'). Assessment of severity depends upon clinical, biochemical and radiological parameters.

The Truelove–Witts index (Table 1) is widely used and with the additional measurement of CRP, which responds more rapidly than ESR, recognising a patient with acute severe colitis should be possible. Predicting outcomes is less easy, but a CRP of > 45 mg/l, and more than three liquid stools per day on the third day of treatment, predict an 85% colectomy rate. Surgery is normally performed after 10–14 days of aggressive medical management without signs of improvement.

Toxic dilatation of the colon has a poor response rate to medical treatment and frequently requires surgery. All patients should be regularly assessed and combined management with the surgeon is optimal.

Treatment of acute severe colitis

1. Hospitalise severe cases and exclude infection.
2. Intravenous hydrocortisone 100 mg q.d.s. (oral prednisolone has variable absorption).
3. Food and water as normal. Additional parenteral feed only if malnourished or unable to eat. Blood transfusion if necessary.
4. Aminosalicylates (ASA compounds) probably offer little additional benefit to adequate doses of hydrocortisone but are often used orally and topically.
5. Heparin prophylaxis for deep vein thrombosis and pulmonary embolism – particularly with a raised platelet count, and immobility.

Anti-diarrhoeals should be avoided as

they do nothing to expedite remission, mask progress, and may make toxic dilatation more likely. Opiate analgesics may have a similar effect and NSAIDs should be avoided for the reasons outlined above. Antibiotics should be used for confirmed infection such as with *Salmonella* but otherwise routine use of antibiotics is unhelpful.

Cyclosporin has been used and may reduce the colectomy rate initially but studies have suggested that this largely defers rather than prevents colectomy. Full anticoagulation with unfractionated heparin has also been used, but there are insufficient data to support its routine use at present.

The decision to move to colectomy is extremely difficult for both the clinician and the patient. It is probably made easier by frequent attendance to the patient and open discussion of management options. There are immediate indications for colectomy and these include intractable haemorrhage and perforation. Medical therapy is much less likely to succeed if there has been no improvement following 7 days of adequate therapy and most clinicians recommend surgery at between 10 and 14 days following initiation of therapy if there has been no response. Patients are often young, and discussion with the family throughout treatment makes the decision to proceed to surgery more straightforward.

It is reassuring sometimes for the patient to know that the response following colectomy is usually dramatic and that a feeling of well-being returns promptly. It is also worth the physician attending the operating theatre to see the colon at the time of colectomy as he or she may find it reassuring to see how diseased the colon appears.

Treatment of moderately severe attacks
This is usually undertaken as an outpatient and most commonly in patients with previously diagnosed UC. In new presentations, ASA compounds can be started immediately whilst awaiting stool cultures, and corticosteroids can be added at a later stage once infection has been excluded. ASA compounds dosing should be increased to optimal levels such as mesalazine 800 mg t.d.s or higher. Failure to respond to this following 2 weeks of treatment is usually an indication to start corticosteroids such as oral prednisolone 40 mg per day. Failure to give adequate doses results in poor outcomes and may make subsequent treatment more difficult. Once an improvement is achieved, reduction of the dose should not be too rapid as this makes a subsequent flare-up more likely, and reduction of prednisolone by 5 mg per week (which therefore takes 8 weeks to stop the steroid) is a reasonable approach. Concurrent use of topical steroids or ASA may also help to reduce the tenesmus which frequently accompanies a flare.

Maintenance therapy of distal disease (proctitis/left-sided disease)
Ideally, distal disease should be treated with topical therapy. There are both steroid and ASA preparations available either as suppositories for proctitis or enemas and foam for slightly more extensive disease. Enemas are slightly more inconvenient to use as they are of higher volume than the foams, but they may spread more proximally, treating up to the splenic flexure. It is usual to use steroid preparations first and retain ASA preparations for more resistant disease because they tend to be more expensive.

Topical preparations can be used intermittently to control flares, or oral therapy can be used continuously to try to prevent recurrence. Occasionally, proctitis can be very resistant to therapy, requiring long-term topical therapy or oral corticosteroids. Cyclosporin and bismuth enemas have also been used with some success for resistant proctitis.

Maintenance therapy of more extensive disease (disease beyond the splenic flexure)
All patients with ulcerative colitis should be on an ASA preparation to reduce relapse rates and this probably reduces the risk of developing colon cancer in the longer term. Choosing among the different preparations available (Table 2) is usually straightforward, but some patients are intolerant of various preparations and others may need to be tried. Patients with particular problems with their joints should be started on sulphasalazine.

There are a number of patients who despite ASAs have recurrent flare-ups requiring courses of steroids. Azathioprine in a dose of 2 mg per kg can be introduced with a tapering dose of steroids and maintained with a small dose of prednisolone such as 5 mg a day. This has been shown to be helpful in reducing exacerbations. However, azathioprine is associated with a number of potentially serious adverse effects including bone marrow suppression, hepatitis and pancreatitis. Prior to initiating this therapy, it is imperative to warn patients of these potential adverse effects. Instruct them that blood monitoring is required in order to try to detect these reactions early and that benefit from azathioprine does not begin for 6 weeks after initiation of therapy and is not maximal until 3 months of treatment have been given.

Table 1 **Severe ulcerative colitis: Truelove–Witts index**

	Value
Diarrhoea with blood in stool	> 6/day
Temperature	> 37.5°C
Haemoglobin	9 g/dl or less
ESR	> 30 mm/h

Table 2 **ASA compounds available for ulcerative colitis**

Drug	Preparation	Method of release
Sulphasalazine	5-ASA linked to sulphapyridine	Bacterial cleavage in colon
Asacol (e-c mesalazine)	5-ASA pH-dependent coating	Dissolves at pH 7 or higher
Salofalk (e-c mesalazine)	5-ASA pH-dependent coating	Dissolves at pH 6 or higher
Pentasa (m-r mesalazine)	5-ASA in semipermeable membrane	Timed release of drug at luminal pH 6 or higher
Dipentum (olsalazine)	A dimer of two 5-ASA molecules, linked by azo bond	Colonic bacteria cleave azo bond
Colazide (balsalazide)	5-ASA linked to 4-aminobenzoyl-3-alanine	Colonic bacterial cleavage

e-c = enteric-coated; m-r = modified-release

ULCERATIVE COLITIS III

NUTRITION

Unlike in Crohn's disease, specific nutritional therapy does not appear to be beneficial in ulcerative colitis. However, up to half of patients may be malnourished and dietary intake is often reduced during an exacerbation, at a time when energy and protein losses are high. Enteral supplementation is the ideal and it is only rarely necessary to feed patients parenterally. It is worth considering preoperatively how long the patient will be unable to eat after the operation, and if this is more than 5 days in a malnourished patient then total parenteral nutrition should be instituted.

SURGERY

Indications – immediate

The indications for surgery are acute severe colitis not responding to medical treatment, toxic dilatation and/or perforation and haemorrhage.

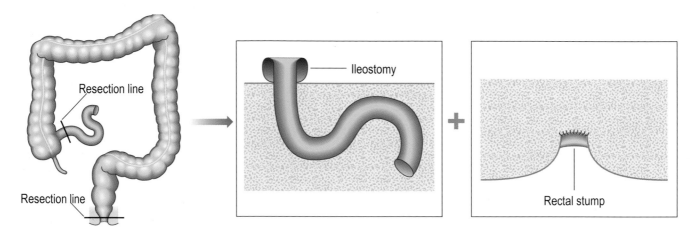

Fig. 1 **Colectomy and ileostomy.**

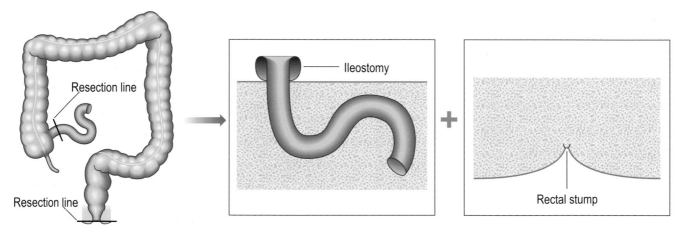

Fig. 2 **Panproctocolectomy and ileostomy.**

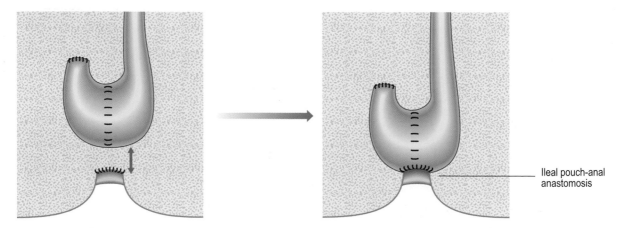

Fig. 3 **Ileal pouch–anal anastomosis.**

1. **Acute severe colitis.** This is characterised by tachycardia, pyrexia, leucocytosis and hypoalbuminaemia. The abdomen may be tender to palpation. Even with optimal medical and surgical treatment, the mortality is still about 5%.

2. **Toxic dilatation.** The patient will have similar symptoms to those above but the abdomen is also distended and straight abdominal X-ray shows colonic dilatation. The danger lies in the increased risk of perforation which increases mortality to up to 40%. Many of the clinical signs may be absent if the patient is on high-dose steroids and therefore diagnosis may be delayed.

3. **Haemorrhage.** Massive haemorrhage is an infrequent complication and is often associated with fulminant colitis and/or toxic megacolon.

Surgery in such patients is extremely high risk and a successful outcome depends upon careful preoperative preparation. This involves:

- correction of any fluid and electrolyte imbalance
- correction of anaemia
- prophylaxis against thromboembolic disease: low molecular weight heparin and compression stockings
- perioperative antibiotic prophylaxis: usually a cephalosporin plus metronidazole or augmentin
- increasing the dose of steroids, which most patients will already be taking, to cover the perioperative period.

Surgery in the acute case is primarily to save life. Invariably the patient will have pancolitis, although in some patients the rectum may be relatively free of disease. It is usually necessary to remove the entire colon (total colectomy) and bring out an ileostomy. If possible, part or all of the rectum is preserved, giving the patient the option of a restorative procedure at a later date (Fig. 1).

Indications – elective

The indications for elective surgery fall into two groups:

1. **Failure or complications of medical treatment.** There will often be an inadequate response to medical treatment, such as chronic diarrhoea, urgency or anaemia. Such patients will often relapse when systemic steroids are discontinued and may therefore start to develop the side-effects of prolonged steroid use and be intolerant of immunosuppression. This is particularly important in children and adolescents where failure to thrive and growth retardation may be present. Some patients will simply fail to comply or will develop side-effects from medication.

2. **Complications of chronic disease**:
   a. Dysplastic or malignant change. The annual incidence of malignancy may be as high as 2% in patients who developed colitis at a young age and have had the disease for over 10 years.
   b. Growth retardation in children; malnutrition in adults.
   c. Extracolonic manifestations of disease. Up to 30% of patients will have at least one extracolonic manifestation and this may contribute to the decision to proceed with surgery.

The aim of surgery in the elective situation is to rid the patient of disease. This invariably requires a proctocolectomy. By removing the 'offending organ', the patient will effectively be cured. There will no longer be a requirement for medication, the cancer risk will be removed and the extracolonic manifestations will often improve, although some (such as sclerosing cholangitis) may progress. Growth and development will usually return towards normal.

Panproctocolectomy and ileostomy (Fig. 2) is the traditional procedure for ulcerative colitis. It achieves the aim of eradicating the disease but does leave the patient with a permanent stoma. This procedure may be preferable in patients who are not suitable for sphincter-saving surgery (see below). It is likely to be the procedure of choice in elderly patients or in those with weakened sphincters, and in those with carcinoma in the lower rectum.

Proctocolectomy with ileal pouch–anal anastomosis (Fig. 3) is now the procedure of choice for many patients with ulcerative colitis. It has the advantage of both removing the disease and avoiding a permanent ileostomy. In this procedure the colon and rectum are removed down to the pelvic floor. A pouch of ileum is fashioned into the shape of the letter 'J' and is sown onto the lower rectum. The pouch acts as a reservoir to store effluent. On average, the patient may need to evacuate about five times during the day and once at night. Many patients find this preferable to the presence of a stoma.

The procedure is technically demanding and is not without complications. The most common early complications are small bowel obstruction and sepsis, which occur in up to 50% of patients. The most common late complication is 'pouchitis' where the ileal pouch becomes inflamed, with the resulting symptoms of urgency and the passage of frequent, loose, bloody stools. Such patients usually improve with metronidazole. Other long-term problems include poor pouch function and chronic sepsis.

Ulcerative colitis

- UC is an inflammatory condition, of unknown aetiology, where inflammation is limited to the colon
- Inflammation is limited to the mucosa so fistulae and abscesses are unusual.
- Patients typically present with bloody diarrhoea.
- Acute severe colitis requires hospitalisation and aggressive medical therapy, but despite this a proportion of patients will go on to require colectomy.
- Medical treatment is aimed at gaining and maintaining remission.
- Colectomy removes the disease and is a cure.

CROHN'S DISEASE I

DEFINITION

Crohn's disease was first described in 1932. It is a chronic inflammatory condition of unknown aetiology that can affect any part of the GI tract from the mouth to the anus but which predominately affects the terminal ileum and colon. The inflammation is transmural and may result in fistulae. Other systems may be affected such as eyes, skin and joints.

EPIDEMIOLOGY

Peak age of presentation is in the late twenties although it may present in childhood and older adults. The incidence is lower than for ulcerative colitis (UC) and is 2–6:100 000 with highest values in North West Europe, North America and Australia and lower incidences in Japan and Greece. The incidence has risen but has probably reached a plateau.

There is a strong family tendency with first-degree relatives of patients with Crohn's disease having a 35 times relative risk of developing the condition. This is a stronger association than for relatives of patients affected with UC. There is high concordance amongst monozygotic twins and there is felt to be a greater genetic influence in the development of Crohn's disease compared to UC. Inheritance of the predisposition to develop Crohn's disease is probably polygenic but recently the NOD2 gene has been identified and is associated with the development of Crohn's disease.

Although the aetiology is unknown, various observations have been made, such as sufferers tending to be brought up in an urban environment, increased intake of refined sugars prior to developing the disease, lower intake of fruit and vegetables and use of the oral contraceptive pill. In distinction to UC, smoking confers a two-fold increase in the risk of developing Crohn's disease. *Yersinia enterocolitica* can cause an illness similar to Crohn's disease but is not thought to be responsible for the condition itself. Measles virus particles have been found to be present in Crohn's disease tissue and *Mycobacterium paratuberculosis* causes a disease similar to Crohn's disease in cattle (Johne's disease) and has been postulated as the causative agent in

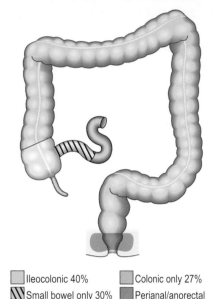

Ileocolonic 40% Colonic only 27%
Small bowel only 30% Perianal/anorectal only 3%

Fig. 1 **Sites of involvement at presentation.**

Crohn's disease. Compelling evidence for either of these agents is still missing, but it would appear that an infection in a host genetically predisposed to the disease will prove to be the cause.

NATURAL HISTORY

Presentation

Symptoms are increased stool frequency, passing loose stools, with blood if there is colonic involvement, and abdominal pain. Weight loss and systemic upset are common. The majority of patients present with ileocolonic or small bowel disease alone (usually terminal ileum) (Fig. 1). The location has an effect on subsequent management and outcome but does not appear to affect the overall mortality related to Crohn's disease, which has been reported as high as 6% but has now undoubtedly fallen and is probably no different from that in the general population.

Clinical course

With aggressive medical management of patients with Crohn's disease, the proportion requiring surgery is falling but has been as high as 90% for patients with ileocolonic disease, 65% for small bowel disease alone and 50% for those with colonic Crohn's. The bowel wall thickening and fibrosis that occur in Crohn's disease make toxic megacolon rare. The disease can behave in an indolent fashion

with one or two minor flare-ups followed by long periods of remission; this is usually in patients who have fibrostenotic lesions of the small bowel. More aggressive disease with raised acute phase reactants and an inflammatory mass have relapse rates of 30% per year. Smoking, the oral contraceptive pill, non-steroidal anti-inflammatory drugs and bacterial infections can all induce a flare-up and should be avoided.

The course of the disease does not appear to be altered by surgery, and reoperation rates are ~ 50% at 5 years, whilst 75% will have endoscopic evidence of disease activity at the anastomotic site at 1 year. Cessation of smoking definitely reduces the risk of post-surgical recurrence but ASA compounds (aminosalicylates) and immunosuppression with azathioprine or 6-mercaptopurine may also have an effect.

DIFFERENTIAL DIAGNOSIS

In young adults or children who present with abdominal pain and diarrhoea, the differential diagnoses include irritable bowel syndrome, other inflammatory bowel diseases (UC or Behçet's disease) and intestinal infections such as tuberculosis. In the older adult, colon cancer also enters the differential, and small bowel lymphoma can cause a right iliac fossa mass and deformity of the terminal ileum (Table 1).

INVESTIGATIONS

The aim of investigation is to confirm the diagnosis and assess disease location, extent and severity. Initial investigations include a full blood count, measurement of ESR and CRP level, biochemistry and liver function tests. Stool culture is used to exclude an infective cause and serol-

Table 1 **Differential diagnosis of terminal ileal Crohn's disease**

Infections/inflammation
Appendiceal abscess
Ileocaecal tuberculosis
Yersinia enterocolitica
Amoebiasis with an amoeboma
Mycobacterium avium-intracellulare and CMV (in AIDS)
Pelvic inflammatory disease
Behçet's disease
Neoplastic
Carcinoma of the caecum/terminal ileum
Lymphoma
Ovarian tumours

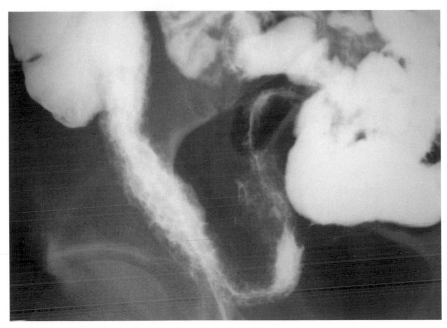

Fig. 2 **X-ray showing abnormal terminal ileum in Crohn's disease.**

White cell scanning is useful in determining disease extent and may be particularly helpful in patients with minor disease (Fig. 4). MR scanning of the pelvis can be helpful in delineating perianal disease.

Endoscopy

Because the majority of patients have terminal ileal disease which is often inaccessible by colonoscopy, endoscopic examination is not always helpful. In patients with upper GI symptoms, the characteristic gastric antral ulceration of Crohn's disease may be seen, and in Crohn's disease affecting the colon, colonoscopy may demonstrate patchy inflammation with areas of intervening normal mucosa ('skip' lesions), ulceration and strictures. The procedure also allows samples to be taken for histology.

Histology

Neutrophils invade crypts and cause a cryptitis as in ulcerative colitis. The intestine ulcerates over a lymphoid follicle and macrophages and monocytes migrate to the area and can change their morphology to epithelioid cells which are non-phagocytic. Macrophages and monocytes fuse to form multinucleate giant cells, which are surrounded by plasma cells and fibroblasts to form the hallmark of Crohn's disease – the granuloma. The absence of granulomas does not preclude the diagnosis of Crohn's disease. Inflammation is transmural.

ogy is helpful for excluding *Yersinia* infection. Blood cultures should be taken in the pyrexial patient. In patients who present with systemic upset, diarrhoea and a right iliac fossa mass, CRP will be elevated, and barium follow-through studies are indicated. In those with obstructive intestinal symptoms who may have a fibrostenotic variant of the condition, small bowel studies are indicated, whilst inflammatory markers are often normal. In those with features of a colitis (bloody diarrhoea and pain), lower intestinal endoscopy is likely to be most diagnostically useful.

Radiology

Small bowel radiology with either small bowel follow-through examinations or, preferably, small bowel enemas, can reveal mucosal oedema, aphthous ulceration, bowel wall thickening and strictures. A 'cobblestone' appearance occurs when transverse and longitudinal ulceration separates areas of more normal mucosa (Fig. 2). Enterocolic and entero-

cutaneous fistulae may also be seen between the terminal ileum and the colon (Fig. 3). In advanced cases, partial intestinal obstruction can be seen with proximal intestinal dilatation above a stricture, and occasionally complete obstruction is seen where there is no passage of barium through a stricture (Fig. 1, p.8).

Barium enema is often used in conjunction with colonoscopy as it outlines affected areas and fistulae, and barium can often be refluxed into the terminal ileum to review this area. Crohn's disease varies in severity but rarely in extent, so repeated radiology is unnecessary unless symptoms change.

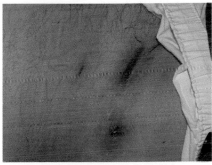

Fig. 3 **Enterocutaneous fistulae in Chrohn's disease.**

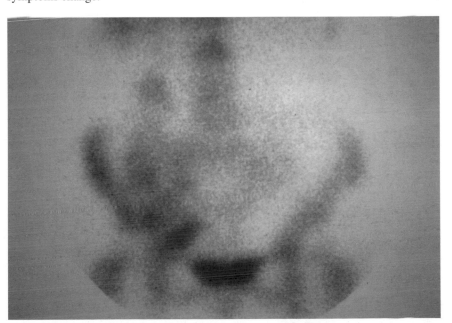

Fig. 4 **White cell scan of Crohn's disease showing activity in the right iliac fossa.**

CROHN'S DISEASE II

ASSOCIATED CONDITIONS / COMPLICATIONS

The associations with eye and joint problems are similar to those seen in UC. Erythema nodosum is more common in Crohn's disease (Fig. 1), whereas pyoderma gangrenosum is more frequently seen in ulcerative colitis. Malabsorption and bacterial overgrowth due to either stasis or fistulae can occur. Mild liver abnormalities are common but serious liver disease is rare. There is an increased risk of developing colon cancer but this appears to be less marked than in UC.

Perianal disease is common with perianal skin tags a frequent finding. Abscesses develop in the anal glands between the internal and external anal sphincters and may track in various directions causing fistulous communications (Fig. 2). Fistulae that develop in front of a horizontal line through the anus with the patient in the lithotomy position communicate in a straight line with the gut, whilst those posterior to this line have an indirect course (Fig. 3).

Because the inflammation in Crohn's disease is transmural, blind-ending tracts can occur which develop into abscesses around areas of disease activity such as in the right iliac fossa. If the tract develops adjacent to another hollow organ or to skin, a fistula can develop. These fistulous communications can be asymptomatic when between lengths of small bowel and do not require treatment, or can cause a series of symptoms:

- marked diarrhoea when enterocolic
- dysuria and pneumaturia when enterovesical
- persistent vaginal discharge when rectovaginal
- chronic discharge of mucus or pus from the skin when enterocutaneous.

They imply areas of active inflammation and chronic sepsis.

TREATMENTS

Terminal ileal disease

Various options are available to control an exacerbation of disease which is limited to the terminal ileum. Delivery systems of ASA compounds tend to mean that the drug is released and is therefore active distal to the terminal ileum. Modified-release mesalazine (Pentasa) is released in the small bowel and has an effect in this area. Corticosteroids are effective but have unwanted side-effects that can be lessened by the use of budesonide, which is released in the terminal ileum and has a high first-pass metabolism in the liver. Dietary treatment with elemental diets (liquid low-residue diets which are adequate nutritionally, readily absorbed and require little or no digestion) may be as effective as corticosteroids in controlling flare-ups, does not have the adverse effects associated with steroids and may be used in conjunction with steroids. Unfortunately, these diets are generally felt to be unpalatable by patients, who often have difficulty tolerating them for the 6 weeks that are required for them to be fully effective.

Maintenance therapy is with ASA compounds and in those who have difficulty discontinuing steroids, immunosuppression with azathioprine along the same lines as in UC is used. Infliximab is a new monoclonal antibody that inhibits the effects of the proinflammatory cytokine tumour necrosis factor α. It appears most useful in patients with refractory Crohn's disease that is not responsive to corticosteroids and azathioprine and in patients with persistent fistulous disease.

Colonic disease

This is treated in a similar fashion to UC, with ASA compounds, corticosteroids and immunosuppression. Dietary treatment appears not to be effective.

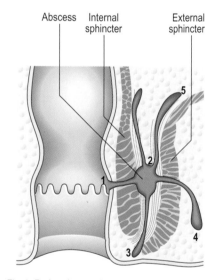

Fig. 2 **Paths of extension and classification of peri-rectal abscesses: 1 cryptoglandular; 2 intersphincteric; 3 perianal; 4 ischiorectal; 5 supralevator.**

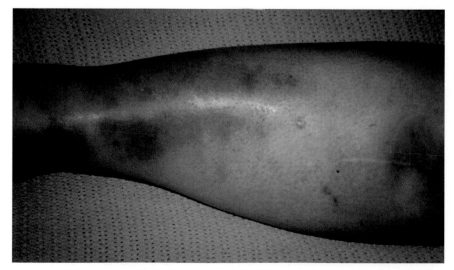

Fig. 1 **Erythema nodosum on the shin.**

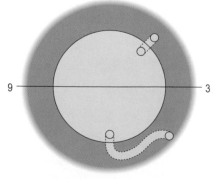

Fig. 3 **Relations of internal and external openings of fistulae-in-ano (patient in the lithotomy position). Behind the 9–3 line, the internal opening is in the 6 o'clock position.**

Abscesses

Metronidazole given as a suppository may be effective in treating perianal sepsis but often incision and drainage are required. Half will close and heal spontaneously, whilst the other 50% will develop into a fistula.

Fistulae

A fistula is an abnormal communication between two epithelial surfaces. Local treatment with metronidazole may help. Immunosuppression with azathioprine closes a small percentage of fistulae and may reduce the risk of further fistula development. Infliximab improves or closes up to 50% of fistulae. Surgical treatment, if necessary, must avoid damage to the external anal sphincter. Subsphincteric and low trans-sphincteric fistulae can be laid open, whereas higher fistulae may require drainage via a seton. This is a piece of suture-like material that is tied through the fistula and around the anal margin to allow permanent drainage.

SURGERY

Because Crohn's disease is a transmural disease, patients are at a higher risk of perforation and intra-abdominal abscess, but are less likely to develop toxic megacolon. A successful outcome once again revolves around good preoperative preparation. Particular emphasis must be placed upon correction of fluid and electrolyte imbalance, correction of anaemia and treatment of sepsis.

Indications for surgery

Failure of medical treatment. This may be an inadequate response to treatment, the development of treatment-related complications or growth retardation in children which may be due to the disease itself, poor nutritional intake and/or malabsorption. Surgical intervention before the end of puberty may allow some catch-up in growth.

Intestinal obstruction. Whilst inflammatory episodes tend to respond well to medical treatment, the development of fibrous strictures or fistulae usually requires surgical intervention. Whilst the vast majority of strictures are located within the small bowel or ileocolic areas, it is important to note that strictures may be multiple and affect more than one area of the gastrointestinal tract.

Fistula and/or abscess formation. Intra-abdominal abscesses will require surgical drainage and resection of the affected bowel.

Carcinoma. There is a reported increase in the incidence of carcinoma in patients with Crohn's disease. As the presentation of both diseases may be similar, the development of malignancy is usually confused with an exacerbation of Crohn's disease and initially treated as such.

Diagnosis is therefore frequently delayed and prognosis poor.

Surgical management

There is now good evidence to show that the risk of developing further Crohn's disease is not influenced by the presence of microscopic disease at the resection margins. Additionally, up to 50% of patients undergoing surgery for Crohn's disease will require a further resection at some future date. The message to surgeons therefore is to be conservative and avoid resecting bowel if at all possible.

Two situations are usually encountered at elective operation. In the first, the bowel is inflamed or involves a fistula. In this situation the area of affected bowel will require excision. Usually, the area involved will be the terminal ileum and this will be dealt with by either a segmental resection or limited right hemicolectomy (Fig. 4). In the second situation the patient has obstructive symptoms owing to a post-inflammatory fibrous stricture. Such strictures are frequently multiple and may occur at the site of a previous resection and anastomosis. The technique of stricturoplasty involves opening the stricture longitudinally and sewing it transversely (Fig. 5). Although the diseased segment is not removed, the obstructive symptoms are relieved in almost all patients, with symptomatic recurrence in just over 20% at 4 years.

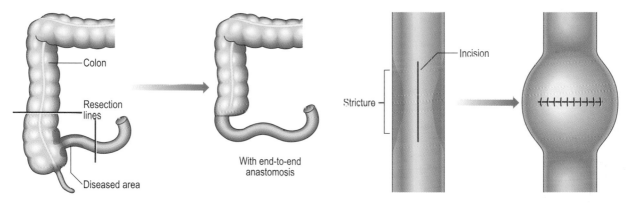

Fig. 4 **Limited right hemicolectomy.**

Fig. 5 **Stricturoplasty.**

Crohn's disease

- Crohn's disease is an inflammatory condition of unknown aetiology that may affect any part of the GI tract.
- Transmural inflammation makes abscess formation and fistulae more common than in ulcerative colitis.

- Diarrhoea, pain and an inflammatory mass in the right iliac fossa are characteristic.
- Bloody diarrhoea tends to occur only when the colon is affected.
- Medical therapy is aimed at controlling exacerbations and maintaining remission.

- Surgical treatment is frequently necessary but recurrence after surgery is the norm.
- Surgical resection, if necessary, should be minimised to prevent significant bowel loss.

INFECTIVE DIARRHOEA

BACTERIA

The proximal small bowel has low bacterial colonisation levels of 10^4/ml, and is protected from increased colonisation by a combination of gastric acid, intestinal motility and bile. The colon has concentrations of 10^{11}/ml of predominately anaerobic organisms. During an episode of infectious diarrhoea the normal flora is replaced by that of the pathogen.

Bacteria exert their effect either by producing a toxin which produces a secretory diarrhoea or by direct mucosal invasion which causes an inflammatory diarrhoea, or by a combination of the two.

Toxigenic organisms

Cholera

This is the classic form of a secretory diarrhoea which has caused pandemics over the last two centuries. Its clinical effect is due solely to the toxin *Vibrio cholerae* produces, which comprises a mucosal-binding portion (B) and an adenylate cyclase-activating portion (A) which stimulates the secretion. 15–20 l of watery stool may be produced per 24 hours, causing profound dehydration. Treatment is aimed at maintaining adequate hydration.

Escherichia coli

A number of pathogenic types of *E. coli* are described:

- enterotoxigenic (ETEC) exert their effect by producing a toxin which induces small bowel secretion
- enteropathogenic (EPEC) are adherent and cause a watery diarrhoea
- enteroinvasive (EIEC) invade the small bowel mucosa and cause a dysentery-like illness
- enterohaemorrhagic (EHEC) may produce a toxin which causes a bloody diarrhoea and is associated with haemolytic–uraemic syndrome in children.

Clostridium difficile

Approximately 20% of antibiotic-associated diarrhoea is caused by toxigenic *C. difficile*. The majority of cases follow the use of antibiotics, particularly clindamycin, cephalosporins and ampicillin/amoxycillin, and cause a colitis, whilst cases not associated with previous antibiotic use may occur in severely debilitated patients, those who have had previous surgery, and patients with leukaemia.

C. difficile may exist as a commensal but exerts its effect by producing toxins. These are enterotoxic (A) and cytotoxic (B). The diagnosis is made by the detection of toxin in the stools. Treatment of mild cases is supportive, with rehydration and discontinuation of the relevant antibiotic. More severe cases may require antibiotic treatment with oral vancomycin or metronidazole, and the most serious episodes can be complicated by toxic dilatation of the colon, which requires corticosteroids or even surgery. Despite treatment, a number of cases relapse and may require further therapy (see Fig. 2, p. 3).

Invasive organisms

Shigella

Four *Shigella* groups (A–D) are recognised, but it is group A that is usually responsible for causing dysentery. This is an inflammatory diarrhoea with blood and neutrophils in the stools. The organisms have a degree of acid resistance and transmission via the oral route may occur with only small numbers of bacteria. The clinical features are of crampy lower abdominal pain with fever and small-volume mucoid stools. Episodes may be complicated by arthralgia. Diagnosis requires stool culture. Antibiotics are now advised for any patient with a fever and the drug of choice is ciprofloxacin.

Salmonella

Non-typhoid. Serotypes *enteritidis* and *typhimurium* are the commonest to cause gastroenteritis. The severity of the illness is proportional to the size of the inoculum. Farmyard animals may harbour the organisms. The illness is characterised by crampy abdominal pain and watery diarrhoea which lasts for a few days.

Diagnosis is confirmed by stool culture. Rehydration plus antibiotics such as ciprofloxacin.

Typhoid. Serotypes *typhi* and *paratyphi* cause typhoid fever, which is a systemic illness characterised by fever, headaches and abdominal pain. Diarrhoea is a feature in only 50% but intestinal haemorrhage and perforation may occur. Diagnosis is usually made on blood culture, and similar antibiotic therapy to that used for non-typhoid types may be used.

Campylobacter

C. jejuni causes a gastroenteritis and in more severe cases a colitis. Infection occurs following ingestion of improperly prepared or cooked food. The condition is usually self-limiting, lasting less than a week, and the diagnosis is made following stool culture.

Yersinia

Y. enterocolitica causes a gastroenteritis and in some cases a more persistent ileitis which can lead to diagnostic confusion with Crohn's disease. Diagnosis can be confirmed on culture or serological testing. A reactive polyarthropathy may occur in individuals with HLA-B27. Antibiotic treatment is not usually required but cotrimoxazole may be used.

Intestinal tuberculosis

The majority of cases are due to *Mycobacterium tuberculosis* and occur following ingestion of infected sputum. Infection most frequently affects the terminal ileum or proximal colon and should be suspected in individuals from Asia or those with active pulmonary TB. The lesions may cause ulceration, fibrosis and strictures, and differentiation from Crohn's disease can be difficult. Treatment is with standard antituberculosis chemotherapy but for prolonged duration.

Table 1 **Worms**

Worm	Pathology	Clinical features	Diagnosis	Treatment
Roundworm *Ascaris lumbricoides*	< 20 cm	Abdominal pain, mass effects, obstructive jaundice	Ova in stools	Mebendazole
Whipworm *Trichuris trichoura*	3–5 cm	Abdominal pain, diarrhoea, rectal prolapse	Ova in stools	Mebendazole
Fish tapeworm *Diphyllobothrium latum*	3–10 cm	None/Vitamin B_{12} deficiency	Ova in stools	Niclosamide
Pork tapeworm *Taenia solium*	2–20 cm	None/larval reaction (cysticercosis)	Ova in stools	Niclosamide
Beef tapeworm *Taenia saginata*	5–25 m	Diarrhoea, malnutrition	Ova in stools	Niclosamide

VIRUSES

Viruses account for about a third of diarrhoeal episodes, particularly in children. The rotavirus causes a short-lived episode in infants, which usually just requires rehydration. The Norwalk agent (winter vomiting disease) causes a range of symptoms, including diarrhoea, abdominal cramp and vomiting. Enteric adenoviruses may also cause longer episodes of diarrhoea lasting up to 2 weeks.

PROTOZOA

Giardiasis

Infection due to *Giardia duodenalis* (formerly *lamblia*) is worldwide but particularly prevalent in Eastern Europe and the Rocky Mountains of the USA. Asymptomatic carriage is common but active disease causes diarrhoea and occasionally steatorrhoea. Vitamin B_{12} and folate malabsorption may ensue. The diarrhoea may occur because of the trophozoites simply covering the mucosal surface. There are associations with IgA and IgM deficiency. Diagnosis is best made by duodenal aspiration as stools may be negative in 50%. Treatment is with a single dose of tinidazole.

Amoebiasis

Infection with *Entamoeba histolytica* may result in asymptomatic carriage of cysts or colitis. Transmission occurs by ingesting cysts which, unlike the trophozoites, can exist outside the host. Ulceration results in bloody diarrhoea with occasionally toxic dilatation, colonic perforation and haemorrhage. The disease is often most active in the proximal colon. A fibrous/inflammatory mass may develop and cause obstruction (amoeboma) and hepatic abscesses can develop, sometimes years after initial infection. Demonstration of trophozoites in the stool establishes the diagnosis in 90%; cysts demonstrate carriage. Treatment is with metronidazole.

Cryptosporidia

These small protozoa cause a self-limiting diarrhoeal illness following ingestion of contaminated water. Their importance, along with microsporidia, is in the infection of immunocompromised patients such as those with AIDS, in whom an intractable illness may ensue. Diagnosis may be made by examination of stools, or histology of small bowel biopsies or electron microscopy. Treatment is unnecessary in the immunocompetent.

WORMS (Table 1)

Ascariasis (roundworm)

Infection is worldwide but most prevalent in the tropics. Colonisation of the small intestine by worms of up to 20 cms length occurs following ingestion of embryos which undergo a circuitous route of re-infection back to the gut via the portal vein, liver and lungs – only on their second pass maturing into adult worms. Large masses of worms may cause symptoms by their mass effect such as obstruction, or may produce malnutrition by competing for ingested nutrients. Diagnosis is made by demonstrating ova in the stool, and treatment is with mebendazole.

Whipworm

So named because of its long, whip-like anterior end, there is worldwide distribution of the causative organism, *Trichuris trichiura*, which causes abdominal pain, diarrhoea, anaemia and malnutrition. Diagnosis is made by demonstrating ova in the faeces; treatment is with mebendazole.

Schistosomiasis

This is an infection caused by *Schistosoma mansoni*, *S. japonicum* and *S. haematobium*, which are parasitic flatworms with an unusual life cycle that includes man and a water snail. The worm larvae (cercariae) penetrate the skin of people walking in fresh water containing the infected host snails in the tropics, Asia, and particularly Egypt, where infection occurs in 80% of the population. Eggs layed by the adults migrate through the bowel wall, causing inflammation and polyp formation resulting in bloody diarrhoea. Treatment is with praziquantel.

TRAVELLER'S DIARRHOEA

With worldwide travel now commonplace for both business and tourism, individuals are becoming exposed to organisms that the indigenous populations are used to, but for which the traveller has no immunity. 'Traveller's diarrhoea' groups these organisms together and the causative pathogens will reflect the local prevelance of these organisms (Fig. 1, Table 2). Episodes usually start on the third day and last 2–4 days. Symptoms are characterised by bowel frequency of 4–6 times per day and crampy lower abdominal pain. Episodes are usually self-limiting and do not require specific diagnosis but just supportive measures.

Advice for travellers attempting to avoid an episode of traveller's diarrhoea should include avoiding uncooked/unpeeled food, ice cubes, tap water, and reheated foods. Foods should be cooked to temperatures $> 65°C$, and caution should be shown in swimming. Bacterial prophylaxis with a quinolone such as ciprofloxacin reduces the risk of attacks by up to 85%. Specific treatment may be required if specific organisms are identified.

REHYDRATING AGENTS

Electrolyte/glucose combinations help rehydrate, replace lost electrolytes and supply energy for Na^+/K^+ ATPase.

Table 2 Geographical areas characterized according to risk of traveller's diarrhoea

Low Risk (<8%)
N. America, Northern and Central Europe, Australia, New Zealand
Intermediate risk
Caribbean, North Mediterranean, Israel, Japan, South Africa
High Risk (20-50%)
Latin America, Africa, Asia

Infective diarrhoea

- Diarrhoea kills millions of children each year worldwide.
- Organisms may exert their effect either by local invasion or by release of toxin.
- Rehydrate with glucose/electrolyte solutions.
- Traveller's diarrhoea is usually self-limiting and does not require specific treatment.
- Alternative diagnoses from traveller's diarrhoea should be considered in persistent cases, such as post-infective irritable bowel syndrome and idiopathic inflammatory bowel disease.

MISCELLANEOUS COLITIDES AND OTHER CAUSES OF DIARRHOEA

MICROSCOPIC COLITIS

It is reasonable to include two relatively recently described conditions in this section: collagenous colitis and lymphocytic colitis, which have similar clinical features but differ in their histology.

Collagenous colitis

This is a condition first described just over 20 years ago which predominately affects women (9 : 1) in their middle and later life (athough a quarter of cases may present aged less than 45). The aetiology is unknown but has been associated with NSAID usage and coffee consumption. Various conditions may coexist, such as rheumatoid arthritis, coeliac disease and scleroderma. The condition itself may be associated with a non-inflammatory arthritis. It is being recognised more frequently and may have a prevalence of up to 15 per 100 000.

The clinical features are of a watery diarrhoea which may be nocturnal and associated with crampy abdominal pain. Hypokalaemia may develop. There is a mild degree of inflammation so that changes in ESR and cytokines are minimal.

The sigmoidoscopic appearance is usually normal, and diagnosis depends on histology, which demonstrates an abnormally thick subepithelial collagenous band of greater than 10 μm (normal thickness = 0–3 μm) (Fig. 1). Barium enema examination is normal, so the condition will be missed unless colonic biopsies are taken. Rectal biopsy alone may fail to demonstrate this change as the band is non-continuous and may be most marked in the proximal colon. Patients may respond to salazopyrin, cholestyramine or corticosteroids.

Lymphocytic colitis

This condition has a number of similarities with collagenous colitis and may represent an earlier stage of the same condition. However, the sex incidence is different, with only twice as many cases occurring in women as in men but with similar age of onset and prevalence. The aetiology is unknown but ranitidine and carbamazepine have been associated with the condition. There is watery diarrhoea with a macroscopically normal colon and histol-

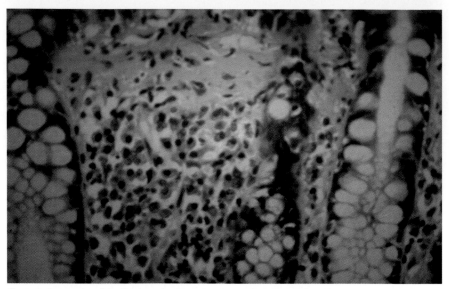

Fig. 1 **Collagenous colitis. Thickened collagen band seen in collapenous colitis.**

ogy showing increases in intraepithelial lymphocytes. There are similar associations with autoimmune diseases and treatment is along the same lines as for collagenous colitis.

RADIATION COLITIS

Following therapeutic irradiation, an acute injury to the gut may occur with inflammation and bloody diarrhoea. This is usually self-limiting.

Delayed damage may occur in around 10% of patients who have received irradiation, usually to the pelvis for malignancy in the prostate, bladder or reproductive tract. Onset occurs with a mean interval of 2 years following treatment. A chronic vasculitis develops with inflammation, stricturing, telangiectases and occasional fistula formation. Treatment of this chronic stage can be difficult but usually begins with ASA compounds (aminosalicylates) and corticosteroids. Bleeding telangiectases may be treated with argon beam photocoagulation or laser therapy.

WHIPPLE'S DISEASE

This is a rare condition that predominately affects middle-aged men and is characterised by intestinal malabsorption with diarrhoea and weight loss, arthralgia and skin pigmentation. The condition may affect many other organs, including the heart with an endocarditis or pericarditis, lungs with pleurisy, and brain with an encephalopathy. The condition is caused by a widespread infiltration of tissues with a small, Gram-positive bacillus – *Tropheryma whippelii*. The small bowel appears thickened and oedematous, and villi are widened and infiltrated by PAS-positive macrophages which phagocytose the bacilli. Previously fatal, this condition is now effectively treated by long courses of antibiotics such as tetracycline or penicillin. Relapse is frequent and progress should be monitored by small bowel biopsy.

SMALL BOWEL LYMPHOMA

The gut is not infrequently involved by extranodal lymphoma but is only rarely the site of a primary lymphoma. When the gut is affected, the small bowel is the second most common site to be affected after the stomach, and patients may present with pain, obstruction or systemic changes of weight loss and anaemia. A mass may be palpable but fever and diarrhoea are relatively uncommon. Lesions complicating coeliac disease are usually of T cell origin and occur in the jejunum, whereas the rest of primary lymphomas are usually of B cell type. Areas of lymphomatous involvement may demonstrate thickened mucosal folds, polypoid mass lesions or mucosal ulceration. Small lesions may be successfully treated by surgical resection alone but adjuvant chemotherapy may be necessary for more extensive lesions following surgical debulking.

α-CHAIN DISEASE (IMMUNOPROLIFERATIVE SMALL INTESTINAL DISEASE – IPSID)

This condition is specifically located in the Eastern Mediterranean area, particularly Iran. The basic aetiology seems to be similar to that of MALT tumours of the stomach in that the condition may be initiated by chronic bacterial antigenic stimulation which results in subsequent malignant change. Chronic malnourishment and unhygienic environs produce a proliferation of immune cells which produce the heavy chain portion of IgA. There is associated suppression of normal IgA production, which may then result in small bowel bacterial overgrowth, which exacerbates the problem. There is a premalignant stage during which prolonged treatment with antibiotics such as tetracycline may result in cure. This is followed, however, by a frankly malignant stage which requires chemotherapy. Clinical features are of abdominal pain, weight loss, diarrhoea and finger clubbing in a young adult from the appropriate geographical area.

SMALL BOWEL BACTERIAL OVERGROWTH

The proximal small bowel has relatively low concentrations of organisms. This situation is maintained by rapid transit of small bowel content, mucous secretion and a lack of stasis. When these mechanisms are inadequate (Table 1), a rise in small intestinal flora occurs that can result in diarrhoea, malabsorption and vitamin deficiency. The protective aspects of intestinal motility and gastric acid production are less effective in the elderly and, consequently, small bowel bacterial overgrowth is more common in the aged and probably under-recognised. The diarrhoea seems to occur as a result of deconjugation of bile salts by bacteria and fat malabsorption. There may be a rise in serum folic acid as this may be produced by gut bacteria.

Diagnosis may be made by documenting an early rise in exhaled hydrogen, owing to small bowel bacterial metabolism, following an ingested carbohydrate load. This test lacks sensitivity and specificity but is easily performed. Use of ^{14}C-xylose as the carbohydrate substrate is more accurate as xylose is completely absorbed in the proximal small bowel and none reaches the colon. Culture of jejunal contents demonstrating $> 10^5$ organisms per ml is the gold standard test but is not routinely performed.

Treatment is aimed at the predisposing condition, and antibiotics such as tetracycline and metronidazole in combination for 14–28 days may be necessary. Relapses are common.

LACTOSE INTOLERANCE

Lactase (a disaccharidase), normally located in the brush border of the small bowel, hydrolyses lactose to glucose and galactose (Fig. 2). In the period following weaning, lactase activity in most populations of the world reduces, such that adults tend to have an acquired lactose intolerance. This tends not to be the case amongst Caucasians in whom the lactase activity persists into adulthood in the majority. In the 10–20% of individuals who are lactose intolerant, the non-absorbed sugars are metabolised by the colonic flora, producing gas, with distension, borborygmi and diarrhoea.

Secondary lactase deficiency may develop following small bowel diseases such as gastroenteritis, malnutrition, coeliac disease and Crohn's disease. If suspected, a trial of dairy-free products is straightforward, but more formal testing may be done with a lactose hydrogen breath test.

DRUGS

The list of drugs that may cause diarrhoea is impressive (Table 2) and a very careful drug history is essential in all patients. This should include not only prescribed medication but also over-the-counter preparations and herbal remedies. The only way to be sure that a drug is not playing a part is to discontinue it. Occasionally patients with psychological problems deliberately abuse laxatives, which may make diagnosis difficult. Phenolphthalein-containing laxatives can be detected by alkalinising stool water, which goes red in the presence of phenolphthalein. Anthraquinone laxatives can be detected by chromatography in urine or stool.

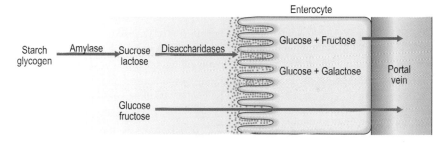

Fig. 2 **Carbohydrate digestion and absorption.**

Table 1 **Conditions that may result in small bowel bacterial overgrowth**

Reduced gastric acid production
Ulcer surgery
Acid suppression therapy
Atrophic gastritis
Stagnation and reduced transit
Small bowel diverticula
Surgical blind loops
Obstruction (strictures, adhesions)
Motility disorders (diabetes, scleroderma)
Fistulas between colon and small bowel

Table 2 **Common drugs that may cause diarrhoea**

- Antibiotics
- Promotility agents – metoclopramide
- Proton pump inhibitors – omeprazole, lansoprazole
- Non-steroidal anti-inflammatory drugs
- Colchicine
- Biguanides – metformin
- Misoprostol
- Cytotoxics
- 5-HT reuptake inhibitors (SSRIs)
- ASA compounds

Miscellaneous colitides and other causes of diarrhoea

- Consider microscopic colitis in a middle-aged woman with watery diarrhoea.
- Colonic biopsy should be performed in all patients with chronic diarrhoea.
- Diarrhoea in a middle-aged man with an extra-intestinal phenomenon such as arthralgia should lead one to consider Whipple's disease.
- Intestinal lymphoma is often a difficult diagnosis to make and may require open surgical biopsy to confirm.
- Small bowel bacterial overgrowth is underdiagnosed in the elderly.
- Lactose intolerance may be detected either following a breath test or by a trial of dairy product avoidance.
- Many drugs have the potential to cause diarrhoea and discontinuation is the only way of excluding them as a cause.

ENDOCRINE, POST-SURGICAL AND LIFESTYLE CAUSES OF DIARRHOEA

THYROTOXICOSIS

Gut disturbance is common in thyrotoxicosis, occurring in approximately 25% of cases. Symptoms are of diarrhoea, colicky abdominal pain and weight loss. The diarrhoea is probably due to a combination of increased small bowel motility and increased mucous secretion via increased cAMP production. The other systemic signs of thyrotoxicosis should be sought – namely tachycardia, tremor, eye signs, brisk reflexes and signs of weight loss.

Gastrinomas

Gastrin-secreting tumours usually occur in the pancreas or duodenum and are associated with persistent peptic ulceration but frequently cause diarrhoea also (see p. 27).

VIPoma

A VIPoma (vasoactive intestinal polypeptide-oma) is a rare functional tumour of the pancreas, producing excess amounts of VIP, which results in severe watery (secretory) diarrhoea, hypokalaemia and hypochlorhydria. The diarrhoea is of large volume, continues during fasting and often results in dehydration. Diagnosis is confirmed by demonstrating an elevated serum VIP concentration in the presence of diarrhoea and frequently a mass in the tail of the pancreas. Functional suppression of the tumour can be achieved with the somatostatin analogue octreotide but surgical excision is the treatment of choice.

Carcinoid syndrome

Tumours secreting 5-hydroxytryptamine (5-HT or serotonin) most commonly occur in the terminal ileum and appendix, but do not produce the syndrome because 5-HT is readily metabolised by the liver. Only when there is metastatic disease in the liver (Fig. 1) or the tumour drainage is not via the portal system (as in bronchial or ovarian carcinoids), does the syndrome occur.

The clinical features (Fig. 2) are of diarrhoea, flushing affecting the chest and head (Fig. 3), bronchospasm, right-sided heart valve lesions and rarely pellagra (due to excessive tryptophan usage, causing wasting, dermatitis, dementia and diarrhoea). Diagnosis depends on demonstrating an elevated 5-HIAA concentration in the urine associated with bulky hepatic metastatic disease or a primary in the lung or ovary.

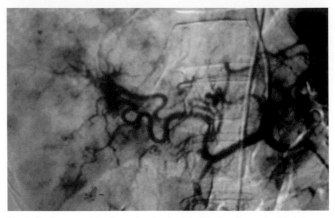

Fig. 1 **Angiogram of the liver showing tumour blushes in carcinoid of the liver.**

Treatment isdirected at controlling, symptoms by debulking the tumour in the liver (either surgically or radiologically), by hepatic artery embolisation or by suppressing 5-HT secretion with octreotide. This often controls both the flushing and diarrhoea, whilst cyproheptadine is most useful in controlling diarrhoea. The tumour obtains its blood supply from the hepatic artery, whereas liver tissue obtains the majority of its oxygen supply from the portal vein. By selective cannulation of the hepatic artery and embolisation of radicals supplying the tumour, tumour tissue necrosis can be achieved with debulking of the tumour, whilst leaving the liver tissue undamaged. This, however, often produces profound metabolic disturbance as there is a surge of 5-HT release.

Diabetes mellitus

Insulin-dependent diabetes is complicated by diarrhoea in about 5% of patients. The stool is usually watery, with occasio-nal steatorrhoea. Symptoms often occur at night and tend to be refractory to therapy. Mechanisms that may contribute include diabetic autonomic neuropathy (where there may be other signs of autonomic dysfunction such as orthostatic hypotension, impotence, neurogenic bladder, pupillary dysfunction, and gustatory sweating), small bowel bacterial overgrowth and abnormal gut motility. Tight diabetic control, antibiotic therapy for bacterial overgrowth, opiates and cholestyramine can all be tried.

Concomitant conditions that occur more frequently in association with diabetes such as coeliac disease and hyperthyroidism should be excluded.

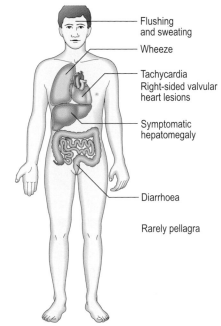

Flushing and sweating

Wheeze

Tachycardia
Right-sided valvular heart lesions

Symptomatic hepatomegaly

Diarrhoea

Rarely pellagra

Fig. 2 **Clinical features of the carcinoid syndrome.**

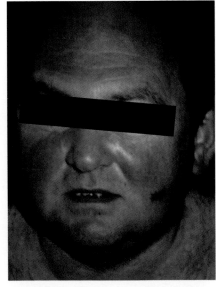

Fig. 3 **Flushing of the face and neck in carcinoid syndrome.**

The oral hypoglycaemic metformin is a common cause of diarrhoea in non-insulin-dependent diabetics, and sorbitol, a sucrose substitute in prepared foods, may also cause diarrhoea (Fig. 4).

POST-SURGICAL CAUSES OF DIARRHOEA

Bile salt diarrhoea

The majority of bile acids are reabsorbed by the terminal ileum as part of the enterohepatic circulation. Following resection of the terminal ileum, non-absorbed bile salts induce a watery diarrhoea by stimulating colonic secretion. The same mechanism may contribute to the diarrhoea in patients with Crohn's disease affecting the terminal ileum. Cholestyramine, an ion-exchange resin, is effective in controlling diarrhoea caused by this mechanism.

Following cholecystectomy, 10–20% of patients complain of mild diarrhoea. The mechanism is not clear but presumably the diarrhoea is a result of disruption of the normal enterohepatic circulation of bile salts. Treatment with cholestyramine or aluminium hydroxide may be helpful.

Short bowel syndrome

The small bowel absorbs approximately 7.5 litres of fluid per day. Following resection, there is considerable capacity for compensation but when more than 1.5m is resected, diarrhoea usually ensues (the normal length is estimated at between 3 and 8 m). The diarrhoea is most marked immediately following surgery and may require intravenous nutritional support whilst compensation occurs. However, it is important to continue enteral feeding during this time as this promotes adaptation. Resection of segments of small bowel can lead to specific nutrient deficiencies (Fig. 5). Resection is most usually performed for Crohn's disease and less frequently for mesenteric infarction and radiation enteritis. The clinical features are of diarrhoea, steatorrhea and macro- and micronutrient deficiency. Features are predictable depending on the amount and site of bowel resected. Moderate resection may allow the patient to remain adequately nourished on a low-fat, high-carbohydrate diet with vitamin supplementation. Calorie intake is often two to three times that required preoperatively. More exten-

sive small bowel resection requires long-term parenteral nutrition. Oral intake may promote a pronounced secretory phase which also results in patients limiting their oral intake so as to avoid volume depletion.

Cholesterol gallstones, liver disease and oxalate kidney stones are more common in patients with short bowel syndrome.

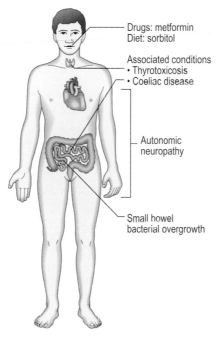

Fig. 4 **Causes of diarrhoea in diabetics.**

Drugs: metformin
Diet: sorbitol

Associated conditions
• Thyrotoxicosis
• Coeliac disease

Autonomic neuropathy

Small bowel bacterial overgrowth

Surgical transplantation of small bowel may be possible in some patients although it has still been performed in only small numbers of patients.

MISCELLANEOUS CAUSES OF DIARRHOEA

Exercise

As recreational exercise becomes more widespread, individuals often observe an urge to defaecate, increased bowel frequency or episodes of watery diarrhoea before, during or after exercise. 'Nervous' diarrhoea, just before a race, occurs in over a third of regular runners and nearly a half experience diarrhoea during a race. Colonic transit times appear to reduce following regular exercise. Reassurance, reducing workload and occasionally prophylactic antidiarrhoeals can be tried.

Alcohol

Alcohol binges often lead to episodes of diarrhoea, possibly owing to decreased gut transit times and inhibition of gut disaccharidases. Chronic alcohol abuse can result in exocrine pancreatic insufficiency, which may be reversible, or chronic pancreatitis. Some beers have naturally occurring high concentrations of salts which act as a cathartic, inducing diarrhoea.

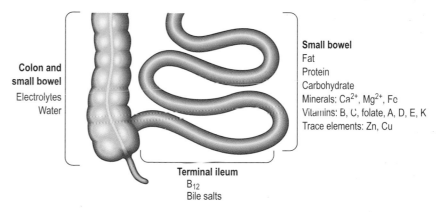

Colon and small bowel
Electrolytes
Water

Small bowel
Fat
Protein
Carbohydrate
Minerals: Ca^{2+}, Mg^{2+}, Fe
Vitamins: B, C, folate, A, D, E, K
Trace elements: Zn, Cu

Terminal ileum
B_{12}
Bile salts

Fig. 5 **Potential components malabsorbed following small bowel resection.**

Endocrine and post-surgical causes of diarrhoea

- Hyperthyroidism is common but diarrhoea as a sole presenting feature is unusual.
- Tumours causing oversecretion of the gut hormones gastrin, VIP and 5-HT can all cause diarrhoea, but are rare.
- Diabetes can be complicated by diarrhoea due to the medication, small bowel bacterial overgrowth and gut dysfunction associated with autonomic neuropathy.
- Diarrhoea associated with the short bowel syndrome is accompanied by micro- and macronutrient deficiency.

THE CLINICAL APPROACH

DEFINITION OF CONSTIPATION

The normal range of bowel frequency is between three times per day and once every 3 days. Anything less frequent than this may be defined as constipation. Patients may also describe straining at stool and passing pellet-like stools (often described as being like 'rabbit droppings'). There may be a sensation of incomplete evacuation. Symptoms persisting for more than 6 weeks may be termed chronic constipation.

PHYSIOLOGY OF DEFAECATION

The urge to defaecate is triggered by distension of the rectum by faeces transported from the sigmoid reservoir by mass motor contractions. Privacy is sought and a squatting position adopted. A Valsalva manoeuvre is often used to increase intra-abdominal pressure in order to promote faecal expulsion. The pelvic floor muscles relax, allowing the pelvic floor to descend. The angle between the anus and rectum is straightened, allowing faecal passage (Fig. 1). Defaecation is a spinal reflex under sympathetic control via the sympathetic chain in front of the aorta and parasympathetics from S2, 3, and 4 to the rectum and internal anal sphincter. The striated muscle of the external anal sphincter is controlled via the somatic pudendal nerve (S2, 3 and 4). When it is inappropriate to defaecate, it is the voluntary contraction of the external anal sphincter that prevents defaecation.

PATHOPHYSIOLOGICAL MECHANISMS OF CONSTIPATION

Because there are so many varied causes of constipation, it is necessary to have a structure for investigating the causes that may be encountered. Of the intestinal causes, one should consider mechanical obstruction – either luminal or due to external compression abnormalities of muscle function, rectal and anal disorders and functional constipation. Extraintestinal causes include drugs, metabolic/endocrine causes, abnormalities of the nervous system (central or peripheral) and psychological causes (Table 1).

HISTORY

As always, taking a thorough history gives the clinician the best chance of making a correct diagnosis and investigating patients appropriately. The individuals most likely to suffer with constipation are young women who have often had their symptoms since their teenage years. If sought, there may also be a family history with mother and sisters being similarly afflicted. Symptoms of abdominal bloating, pain relieved by defaecation, and an alternating diarrhoea and constipation suggest the irritable bowel syndrome. In the older individual who suddenly notices a change in bowel habit associated with symptoms of pain and distension, there may be a mechanical obstruction – stenosing carcinomas of the colon not infrequently cause these symptoms and injudicious use of purgatives in preparation for a barium enema may tip patients into complete obstruction, requiring emergency resection. In these circumstances a barium enema without colonic preparation may give the diagnosis without the risks.

Particular care should be exercised in taking a thorough drug history – patients often forget or omit the non-prescribed treatments they are taking (Table 2). Careful dietary assessment is important because the poor quality of individual diets is often surprising, particularly in regard to intake of dietary fibre. It is worth going through each meal of the day and enquiring what would normally be eaten.

Endocrine or metabolic abnormalities such as hypothyroidism, hypokalaemia and hypercalcaemia may all present with constipation but are often associated with other systemic changes. Neurological causes would usually have constipation as an associated symptom rather than as a presenting feature.

Patients' presenting symptoms may often be masking underlying worries, particularly regarding cancer, and it is worth enquiring about this specifically, as directly addressing the issue and answering the patients' concerns will usually lead to resolution of their symptoms.

EXAMINATION

If a neurological or endocrine cause is suspected, then abnormal clinical signs may be elicited during the general physical examination. The abdominal examination

Table 1 **Causes of constipation**

Idiopathic
Dietary
Inadequate fibre or fluid intake
Intestinal
Luminal tumours (also with external compression)
Strictures (diverticular, ischaemic, infective, inflammatory)
Irritable bowel syndrome
Hirschsprung's disease
Rectocele
Solitary rectal ulcer syndrome/mucosal prolapse
Anismus
Anal fissure
Pseudo-obstruction
Extraintestinal
Spinal cord damage
Parkinson's disease
Cerebrovascular disease
Metabolic/endocrine (hypothyroidism, hypercalcaemia, hypokalaemia)
Drugs

Table 2 **Drugs that may cause constipation**

- Opiates
- Anticholinergics
- Tricyclic antidepressants (anticholinergic side-effects)
- Calcium channel blockers
- Antihistamines
- Diuretics
- Antacids (calcium and aluminium salts)
- Iron
- Chronic laxative abuse

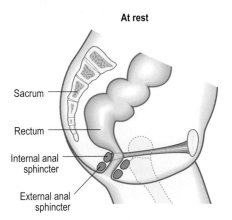

At rest

Sacrum

Rectum

Internal anal sphincter

External anal sphincter

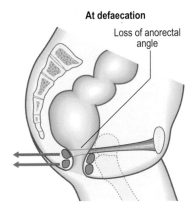

At defaecation

Loss of anorectal angle

Fig. 1 **The pelvis at rest and on defaecation.**

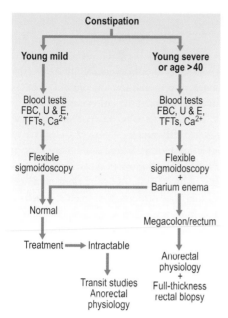

Constipation

Young mild → Blood tests FBC, U & E, TFTs, Ca^{2+} → Flexible sigmoidoscopy → Normal → Treatment → Intractable → Transit studies Anorectal physiology

Young severe or age >40 → Blood tests FBC, U & E, TFTs, Ca^{2+} → Flexible sigmoidoscopy + Barium enema → Megacolon/rectum → Anorectal physiology + Full-thickness rectal biopsy

Fig. 2 **Investigation algorithm for constipation.**

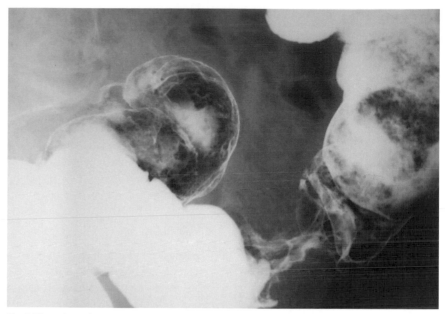

Fig. 3 **Stenosing colon cancer seen on barium enema.**

may reveal masses due to either tumours or distended bowel proximal to an obstruction. Consideration should be given to the patient during rectal examination as this may be painful in the presence of anal fissures or increased anal tone, and it may be kinder to perform rectal examination under sedation prior to flexible sigmoidoscopy in these cases. In the elderly, a loaded rectum suggests faecal impaction, which may be associated with periods of spurious diarrhoea, due to overflow.

Pain in the perineum at the time of defaecation which begins suddenly, particularly when straining to pass a hard stool, and is often associated with a few spots of blood suggests an anal fissure. Intense, episodic, sharp rectal pain which lasts a few moments and then resolves completely is termed proctalgia fugax and may

be associated with symptoms of irritable bowel syndrome.

INVESTIGATIONS (Fig. 2)

Deciding who and how far to investigate is an important clinical skill. In the younger age group where irritable bowel syndrome is common, history, examination and flexible sigmoidoscopy, with a full blood count, serum biochemistry, thyroid function tests and measurement of serum calcium concentration may be all that is necessary. Simple advice regarding diet, physical activity and the condition itself may be effective treatment. It would be inappropriate to perform barium examination in individuals who respond to these measures. In an older age group (patients over 40 years) or in younger patients with a strong family history of colon cancer, particularly at an early age, visualisation by either radiology or colonoscopy should be performed, looking for colonic neoplasia (Fig. 3) – the incidence of which increases with age. Colonic dilatation is

best demonstrated by radiology (Fig. 4).

Colonic transit studies (Fig. 5) and anorectal physiology measurements may be necessary in a small subset of patients such as those with megacolon and in patients with severe intractable symptoms.

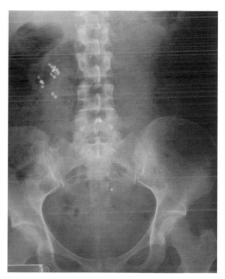

Fig. 5 **Pellets for transit studies seen in right upper quadrant in gut transit study.**

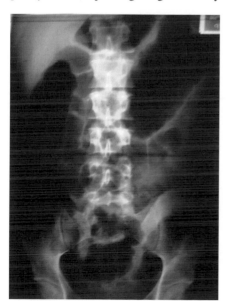

Fig. 4 **Megacolon.**

The clinical approach

- A careful history should include both a dietary evaluation and a drug history–prescribed and over the counter.
- Clearly establish what the patient means by constipation and what symptom he or she would like to have solved.
- Examination may be unhelpful. Rectal examination and, usually, sigmoidoscopy must be performed—if likely to be particularly painful, they can be done under sedation.
- Avoid over-investigation if the symptoms are not severe and there is no evidence of megacolon.
- Psychological factors often play a part and sympathetic management will often be most successful.

RELATED CONDITIONS

SEVERE IDIOPATHIC CONSTIPATION

This condition usually afflicts young women who may have a family history of the condition and whose symptoms began in their teenage years. There is usually abdominal pain and bloating and patients describe infrequent stool passage. Patients have often tried dietary fibre supplements and are usually taking stimulant laxatives at the time of presentation.

Occasionally, patients describe an incredible bowel habit with defaecation every few weeks. Colonic transit time can be established from X-ray images taken at 5-day intervals of a patient who has swallowed radio-opaque pellets. Retention of more than 20% of pellets suggests slow transit constipation. In others, a more normal bowel habit is demonstrated, reflecting patients' perceptions of their bowel habit.

Anorectal physiology studies may show an inability to relax the external anal sphincter when the rectal pressure is increased – such that the rectum is pushing against a 'closed door' (anismus). The aetiology of this is unknown but is probably an acquired condition following persistent suppression of the urge to defaecate.

Treatment

Mild to moderately constipated patients will usually have increased their dietary fibre intake, although some may be helped by formal dietary assessment. Bulking laxatives and then a stimulant suppository such as bisacodyl should be used next. More severe constipation may require enemas, oral stimulant laxatives, or a non-absorbed polyethylene glycol preparation (PEG) (Table 1).

Rarely, surgery is considered. Subtotal colectomy and ileorectal anastomosis has an unpredictable outcome with one-third developing diarrhoea and 10% remaining constipated.

MEGACOLON

If patients complain of constipation since childhood and demonstrate a dilated gut (diameter of the rectum at the pelvic brim exceeds 6.5 cm), adult Hirschsprung's disease should be considered. In this condition, a segment (usually distal) of bowel fails to relax, producing a functional obstruction. Presentation is usually in childhood but the condition may appear in later life. There is aganglionosis with loss of intramural nerve plexuses, which can be demonstrated at histology following a full-thickness mucosal biopsy taken at least 2 cm above the dentate line. Alternatively, rectal physiology studies show a failure of anal relaxation following rectal distension (the recto-anal inhibitory reflex) – its presence excludes Hirschsprung's disease. Surgical resection is required for the rare cases of Hirschsprung's disease.

Acquired megacolon can occur following neurological diseases such as spinal cord injury, Parkinson's disease, diabetic neuropathy, dystrophia myotonica and Chagas' disease, or may be idiopathic.

Treatment should include that of the underlying condition if present, but is aimed at keeping the colon empty.

Acute megacolon can complicate acute severe inflammatory bowel disease and infectious colitis. There is another group in whom megacolon develops acutely, usually with coexisting conditions such as trauma or orthopaedic events; such a development is termed pseudo-obstruction or 'Ogilvie's syndrome'. The clinical features are of marked gaseous abdominal distension developing in an elderly, frail or postoperative patient. Abdominal X-ray shows gaseous distension, and mechanical obstruction is excluded by water-soluble contrast enema (Fig. 1). This may also be therapeutic as treatment is aimed at decompressing the bowel with rectal flatus tubes and enemas. Biochemical abnormalities should be corrected and if this fails decompression by colonoscopy may be required, which will usually be effective. This can be repeated and neostigmine added if necessary.

SOLITARY RECTAL ULCER SYNDROME

Following chronic constipation and straining at stool, particularly in women, mucosa from the anterior rectal wall may prolapse through the anal margin. This results in mucosal damage and ulceration, typically on the anterior rectal wall. Straining at defaecation is accompanied by

Table 1 **Laxatives and their mode of action**

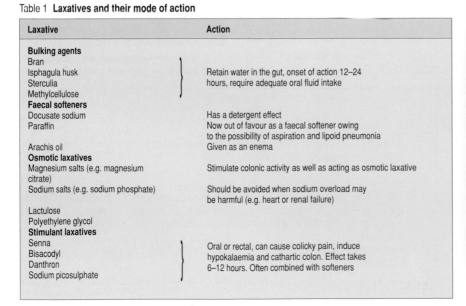

Laxative	Action
Bulking agents Bran Isphagula husk Sterculia Methylcellulose	Retain water in the gut, onset of action 12–24 hours, require adequate oral fluid intake
Faecal softeners Docusate sodium	Has a detergent effect
Paraffin	Now out of favour as a faecal softener owing to the possibility of aspiration and lipoid pneumonia
Arachis oil	Given as an enema
Osmotic laxatives Magnesium salts (e.g. magnesium citrate)	Stimulate colonic activity as well as acting as osmotic laxative
Sodium salts (e.g. sodium phosphate)	Should be avoided when sodium overload may be harmful (e.g. heart or renal failure)
Lactulose Polyethylene glycol	
Stimulant laxatives Senna Bisacodyl Danthron Sodium picosulphate	Oral or rectal, can cause colicky pain, induce hypokalaemia and cathartic colon. Effect takes 6–12 hours. Often combined with softeners

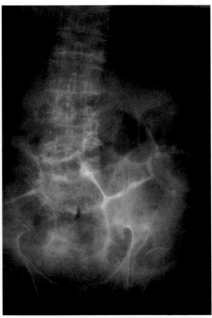

Fig. 1 **Intestinal pseudo-obstruction.**

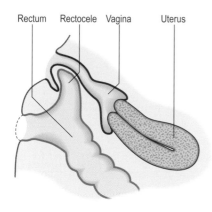

Fig. 2 **Rectocele encroaching on posterior vaginal wall.**

blood and pain. A defaecating proctogram may show the mucosa prolapsing through the anal margin. Histology is characteristic with fibrosis in the lamina propria. Bulking agents and avoidance of straining at stool may help, but surgical fixation may be required.

RECTOCELE

The posterior vaginal wall may prolapse, pulling the anterior rectal wall with it, producing a rectocele (Fig. 2). A rectocele is usually asymptomatic until large, when the patient has a feeling of incomplete evacuation and may need to place a finger in the vagina to empty the rectal sac of faeces. Surgical repair is required.

DESCENDING PERINEUM SYNDROME

Most commonly affecting women following childbirth, the anal margin descends excessively causing closure of the anal canal and obstructed defaecation. Rectal prolapse often results. Observation of the perineum at the time of straining demonstrates the descent of the perineum below a line between the ischial tuberosities. Bulking agents and repair of rectal prolapse may be required.

PERIANAL PAIN

ANAL FISSURES

Characteristic intense anal pain, of sudden onset at the time of passing a hard stool, and often associated with a few drops of blood, is characteristic of an anal fissure. The vast majority occur in the posterior midline or anteriorly, and deviation from these sites raises the possibility of an alternative underlying disease such as Crohn's disease. At the upper margin there may be a hypertrophic anal papilla and, distally, a sentinel pile at the anal verge may be seen.

Anal fissures are usually associated with constipation, and bulking agents and analgesia may allow healing. Glyceryl trinitrate gel and lignocaine gel applied topically will help more severe cases. Lateral sphincterotomy lowers the anal resting pressure and allows healing.

PROCTALGIA FUGAX

A severe pain in the rectum which lasts a few moments and then resolves spontaneously is typical of proctalgia fugax. It is a common symptom, often experienced when individuals are feeling under stress. Reassurance and avoidance of constipation are usually sufficient.

HAEMORRHOIDS

The three major symptoms caused by haemorrhoids or 'piles' are fresh rectal bleeding, local pain and pruritus. Of the mammals it would appear that only man is afflicted with haemorrhoids, although it is unclear why this should be so. It is probably due to straining to pass the low-volume, firm stools that result from a residue-deficient diet. The anal cushions have a rich venous plexus and it is these venous cushions that become enlarged to form haemorrhoids. They characteristically appear in the 3, 7, and 11 o'clock positions (Fig. 3) and may be internal or prolapse through the anal canal (Table 2).

Bleeding and prolapse may be made worse when the patient attempts to pass hard stools and if attempts to defaecate are made before a natural call to stool. The bleeding typically occurs after stool has been passed and may be seen on the toilet paper or dripping into the pan. Blood may appear on the surface of the stool but should not be admixed with it. A history of rectal bleeding warrants some further investigation even in the young and should include a sigmoidoscopy.

An explanation and reassurance are necessary for minor haemorrhoids as the natural history of haemorrhoids is for them to come and go, and treatment may not be necessary. Patients should be encouraged to take more fibre in their diets in order to produce softer stools. Banding of the haemorrhoids is an outpatient procedure in which a band is placed onto the exuberant venous plexus. Care must be taken to ensure that the band is above the dentate line, otherwise the patient experiences severe pain and the band requires removal. Injection sclerotherapy can also be performed, but there are reports of erectile dysfunction in men and, if warned of this possibility, most would decline this form of treatment. Surgical excision is required for irreducible haemorrhoids.

Table 2 **Classification of haemorrhoids**

Degree	Symptoms/findings
First	Bleeding, but not prolapsing
Second	Prolapse but reduce spontaneously
Third	Prolapse but require manual reduction
Fourth	Permanently prolapsed

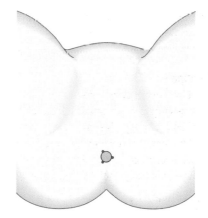

Fig. 3 **Haemorrhoid positions.**

Conditions causing constipation and/or perianal pain

- Constipation-predominant irritable bowel syndrome is a common problem which requires reassurance and advice rather than extensive investigation.
- Anismus is detected by anorectal physiology studies and is best treated by biofeedback techniques.
- Laxatives work by bulking the stool, by acting as a faecal softener, by creating an osmotic gradient in the bowel, or by stimulating the colon.
- Treatment for haemorrhoids includes bulking the stool to keep it soft, reassurance, and therapy to the haemorrhoid only if necessary.

THE CLINICAL APPROACH

The annual incidence of acute upper gastrointestinal haemorrhage is approximately 1 per 1000 adults per year with a mortality in the region of 10%, the majority of deaths occurring in the older age group. This mortality rate appears to have fallen only slightly despite attempts at endoscopic therapy and the development of algorithms attempting to identify high-risk patients.

Management of patients with an acute upper gastrointestinal bleed is slightly different from the management of many other emergencies because initial treatment does not usually depend on establishing a diagnosis. Patients may present with vomiting of frank red blood (haematemesis), which usually does not present a diagnostic conundrum, although swallowed blood from substantial nose bleeds can be misinterpreted as coming from the gastrointestinal tract (GIT). Estimating the volume of blood vomited is difficult and patients may often overestimate the amount. Smaller bleeds can present with vomiting altered blood, which is often described as 'coffee grounds'. The passing of 'melaena' – black sticky stool with a characteristic odour – represents a significant upper GI bleed but may or may not be associated with haematemesis. If the bleed is torrential, degradation of the blood may not have had time to occur and partly altered red blood is passed per rectum (haematochezia).

ASSESSMENT

The first step in management, having been convinced that there has been an upper GI bleed, is to establish the severity and risk to the patient. This requires ongoing measurement of pulse and blood pressure (including looking for the presence of a postural drop in BP, which should warn the clinician that the haemorrhage is larger than may otherwise have been suspected). Peripheral venous access should be gained in minor bleeds or a central venous line should be placed to allow central venous pressure monitoring and maintain good venous access when a larger bleed is suspected. This is particularly so in patients who present with a systolic blood pressure of < 100 mmHg or who have significant comorbidity, particularly liver disease, in whom a variceal bleed is a possibility. Blood should be drawn for haemoglobin estimation, liver function tests, coagulation tests, biochemistry and cross-matching.

Age, shock, comorbidity, diagnosis, major stigmata of recent haemorrhage at endoscopy and rebleeding have all been shown to be independent predictors of mortality and a scoring system has been developed in order to identify these cases (Table 1). Use of this scoring system allows prediction of mortality and rebleeding rates and should allow focusing of monitoring and treatment.

Patients should have their intravascular volume restored with colloid or blood when it becomes available. This should be enough to maintain an adequate blood pressure or raise the haemoglobin above 10 g/dl in the less acute situation.

HISTORY

Having stabilised the patient, more time can be given to taking a history.

A history of recurrent epigastric pain may point towards peptic ulcer disease, and haematemesis following a period of vomiting suggests a Mallory–Weiss tear.

Attention should be given to previous history of haemorrhage, peptic ulcer disease, liver disease, previous surgery including aortic aneurysm repair and bleeding disorders. Note should be taken of current drug therapy, particularly NSAID usage, remembering that NSAIDs may now be obtained over the counter without prescription.

An attempt to quantify alcohol consumption should be made.

EXAMINATION

Having measured the vital signs of pulse and blood pressure, features of chronic liver disease and portal hypertension should be sought. Careful abdominal examination should be performed for the presence of an aortic aneurysm or previous surgery and the mouth inspected for telangiectases. Rectal examination will determine whether melaena is present.

INVESTIGATIONS

The investigation of choice, which also allows therapy to be undertaken, is upper GI endoscopy. This should be undertaken in all patients with an upper GI bleed but the timing of its performance is a more critical question (Fig. 1). Endoscopy of an inadequately resuscitated patient is hazardous and should be avoided; however, in the presence of torrential blood loss, such as may occur with oesophageal varices, resuscitation, diagnosis and treatment must run concurrently. The other patients who should be endoscoped urgently are those with a massive first bleed or a rebleed, elderly patients over the age of 70, and patients with varices. Otherwise, patients should be endoscoped on the next routine list. Unfortunately, patients with the most severe disease who require urgent endoscopy often have the procedure performed by the least experienced endoscopists, out of hours, with nurses who may not be highly trained endoscopy nurses. This is unacceptable because important therapeutic interventions that have an impact on patient outcome can be undertaken during endoscopy.

Following endoscopy, a small percent-

Table 1 **Scoring for acute upper GI haemorrhage**

Component	Score 0	1	2	3
Age	< 60	60–79	> 80	–
Shock	No shock	Tachycardia	Hypotension	–
Pulse rate (bpm)	< 100	>100	–	–
SBP (mmHg)	Normal	>100	< 100	–
Comorbidity	None	–	Ischaemic heart disease	Renal failure Any malignancy
Diagnosis	Mallory–Weiss tear No lesion	All other diagnoses	Malignancy of upper GI tract	–
Stigmata of recent haemorrhage	None	—	Blood in upper GI tract, visible vessel spurting vessel	–

SBP = Systolic blood pressure

age of patients will have no demonstrable cause for their GI bleed. This may occur particularly with a Mallory–Weiss tear and much less frequently with a Dieulafoy lesion.

ENDOSCOPIC STIGMATA OF RECENT HAEMORRHAGE

Certain stigmata are visible endoscopically which are associated with a high chance of rebleeding and usually prompt intervention with endoscopic therapy. When oesophageal varices are discovered, active bleeding, adherent clot or a cherry red spot on a varix indicate active or recent bleeding and sclerotherapy or banding should be undertaken. In Mallory–Weiss tears or ulcers, active bleeding, adherent clot or a visible vessel – usually seen as a black dot in the centre of an ulcer – likewise signify a high risk of rebleeding and warrant therapy.

ENDOSCOPIC THERAPY

Sclerotherapy and banding for oesophageal varices is dealt with in the text on portal hypertension (p. 88).

Sclerotherapy for ulcers, Mallory–Weiss tears and Dieulafoy lesions

Using a similar technique to that of sclerotherapy for oesophageal varices, high-risk lesions can be directly injected via the endoscope, with a sclerosant or an adrenaline solution. Up to 10 ml of 1:10000 adrenaline solution is injected around the perimeter of an ulcer and then directly into the visible vessel. This technique has been shown to reduce rebleeding rates.

CAUSES

Peptic ulcer disease, oesophageal varices (see p. 90), and Mallory–Weiss tears are the commonest causes of acute upper GI haemorrhage. However, other rarer causes

Table 2 Causes of acute upper GI haemorrhage

Common	Less common
Duodenal ulcer	Duodenitis
Gastric ulcer	Oesophagitis
Gastric erosions	Tumours
Mallory–Weiss tear	Hereditary telangiectasia
Oesophageal varices	Aortoduodenal fistula
	Clotting disorder
	Portal hypertensive gastropathy
	Dieulafoy lesions

should not be forgotten, because no obvious cause is found in up to 20% of cases so the differential diagnosis has to be considered frequently (Table 2).

Peptic ulcer disease

Once diagnosis has been established, patients should be started on a high-dose proton pump inhibitor (e.g. omeprazole 40 mg b.d.) for 5 days, which reduces the risk of rebleeding. Careful observation should continue for signs of rebleeding, which include the development of a tachycardia, a fall in BP, or fall in the central venous pressure. Patients with a high-risk lesion should be kept nil by mouth for 48 hours in case surgery is required, and then food should be reintroduced. Patients with low-risk lesions can restart food immediately. Torrential bleeding at endoscopy and

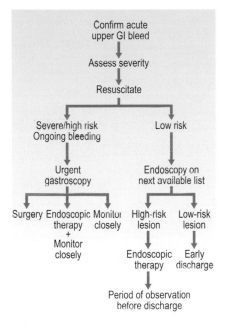

Fig. 1 **Investigation algorithm for acute upper GI bleed.**

rebleeding following endoscopic therapy are an indication for surgery.

Mallory–Weiss tears

The history is characteristic when patients often having consumed alcohol begin to vomit and subsequently have a haematemesis. This is usually relatively mild and stops spontaneously. Because of the violent vomiting, a tear develops in the mucosa of the distal oesophagus or proximal stomach. This can be difficult to see at endoscopy but if it does continue to bleed, injection therapy can be undertaken. Overnight observation in hospital following the endoscopy is all that is required, and a 7-day course of a proton pump inhibitor on discharge.

Dieulafoy lesions

These are calibre-persistent arteries that rise to the surface of the gastric mucosa, erode through it and bleed. They commonly affect elderly men and occur high in the posterior wall of the stomach. They are easy to miss as there is no surrounding ulceration and may just be seen as a bleb. They should be considered when an elderly patient has had a substantial upper GI bleed with an initial examination that reveals no obvious bleeding source. To confirm small lesions to be Dieulafoy, light pressure with an injection needle that has been primed with sclerosant demonstrates arterial bleeding and confirms the diagnosis. It is then necessary to inject sclerosant into the vessel immediately. If not recognised and treated, such lesions result in a significant mortality amongst this age group.

The clinical approach

- Assessment and resuscitation should run concurrently to stabilise the patient.
- Close questioning about drugs, including over-the-counter preparations, is essential.
- Age and comorbidity increase the risk of a bad outcome from an upper GI haemorrhage.
- Endoscopy should be carried out on a resuscitated patient, early if high risk or on the next routine list if low risk.
- Torrential bleeding at endoscopy, or rebleed following endoscopic therapy for peptic ulcers is an indication for consideration of surgery.

IRON DEFICIENCY ANAEMIA

IRON METABOLISM

An average diet provides 10–20 mg of iron/day of which approximately 1 mg is absorbed. Sources include red meat, fish, eggs, cereals and leafy vegetables. The iron in vegetable sources is usually present in the Fe^{3+} state but it is best absorbed in the reduced Fe^{2+} state. Reduction occurs in the stomach with gastric acid and vitamin C. Achlorhydria, previous partial gastrectomy, or a poor intake of dietary vitamin C may reduce absorption. Iron is actively absorbed across the cell wall of the intestinal mucosa, particularly in the proximal small bowel. Hence, damage of this mucosa, which occurs in coeliac disease, often leads to iron deficiency. Once inside the cell, iron is either bound to ferritin and stored within the cell or passed into the circulation bound to transferrin to be transported. Storage occurs in the liver, spleen and bone marrow in the form of ferritin or haemosiderin.

CLINICAL APPROACH

With widely available blood testing, a full blood count revealing a microcytic anaemia is a very common finding in primary health care. This may be simply treated in the community if a cause such as menorrhagia is obvious, or referred for further investigation if the cause is obscure. It is important, however, to confirm iron deficiency in the presence of a microcytic anaemia, and this is best done by measuring serum ferritin – low values confirming iron deficiency. Secondly, remember that iron deficiency has occurred for a reason and that if the clinician is unsure of that reason, then further investigation is necessary.

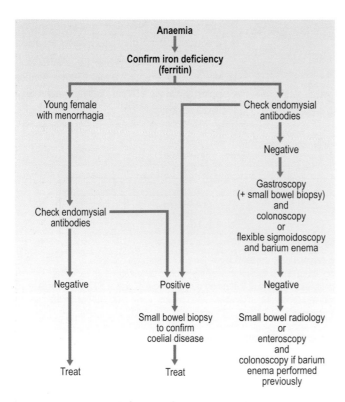

Fig. 1 **Investigation algorithm for iron deficiency anaemia.**

History

The history should include any symptoms that may result from anaemia (tiredness, poor exercise tolerance, breathlessness, worsening angina) although these may be absent in an otherwise fit individual. Teasing out a possible cause is most logically done by considering that for iron to be available for erythropoiesis it must be ingested, absorbed and utilised and that there should not be excessive loss. So dietary intake should be assessed and evidence for malabsorption sought. Evidence for overt gastrointestinal blood loss, or GI symptoms such as dyspepsia, or a change in bowel habit should be sought in all patients, and young women should also be asked about their gynaecological history. Drugs, as ever, are important because GI bleeding is commonly caused by aspirin and NSAIDs. A strong family history of colonic neoplasia should prompt lower GI investigation.

Examination

Examination may reveal evidence of chronic iron deficiency, such as koilonychia, glossitis and angular stomatitis. Telangiectases under the tongue suggest hereditary haemorrhagic telangiectasia; abdominal masses may be due to gastric or colonic neoplasia, and rectal examination should be performed in all to exclude a rectal neoplasm. It is also worth performing a urine dipstick test at presentation because chronic blood loss from the bladder can result in anaemia, particularly in elderly men, and early discovery may prevent a sequence of unnecessary GI investigations.

Investigations (Fig. 1)

Deciding who to investigate is difficult but it is probably appropriate to investigate the GI tract of postmenopausal women, premenopausal women who have light periods, and all men. Investiga-tion ideally should include a serum endomysial antibody test for coeliac disease, colonoscopy and upper GI endoscopy with small bowel biopsy (particularly if the endomysial antibodies are positive). This approach will demonstrate the majority of lesions but approximately 5% will remain obscure following these tests. Small bowel examination is the next logical step, using either barium studies, which are widely available, but have the disadvantage of missing small bowel angiodysplasia (which accounts for the majority of cases of small bowel blood loss) or, preferably, enteroscopy, which allows direct visualisation of the small bowel mucosa.

If still no cause for the GI blood loss is demonstrated and the patient's haemoglobin can be maintained by oral iron supplementation, then it is reasonable to do this. If despite iron the haemoglobin falls, then further investigation can include radioisotope scanning with labelled red cells, but this requires 5–10 ml of GI blood loss per hour, or angiography, which detects 0.5 ml/min. Laparoscopy and on-table endoscopy may help in severe cases.

Faecal occult blood testing (FOBT)

These tests depend on pseudoperoxidase activity in haemoglobin reacting with substrate on guaiac-impregnated paper and producing a colour change. Faeces is placed onto the test paper, with the paper dry or moistened with water. This latter procedure increases the sensitivity of the test but reduces its specificity. Ingested rare red meat and peroxidase-containing vegetables such as broccoli, turnip, cauliflower and radish can lead to false-positive tests, and these foods should be avoided for 3 days prior to testing. Widely studied as a potential screening mechanism for colon cancer, FOBT has a false-negative rate for colonic polyps and cancer of around 40%. This is because:

- tumours bleed intermittently, and so FOBT is recommended on 3 consecutive days
- left-sided colonic lesions tend to bleed less than right-sided lesions and therefore can be missed
- vitamin C and bacterial degradation of haemoglobin by colonic bacteria can reduce the sensitivity of the test.

Oral iron therapy does not appear to have an effect on FOBT.

CAUSES

There are many lesions within the GI tract that have the potential to cause iron deficiency anaemia (Table 1); however, within the older age group, colonic neoplasia (polyps or cancer) and gastric ulcers or gastric cancer are among the commonest and most important causes. A frequently encountered clinical trap is that the upper GI investigations are performed first and a benign lesion such as oesophagitis, which is an unusual cause of anaemia, is thought to be the cause and no lower GI investigations are undertaken, only to find at a later date that a colonic cancer presents.

Gastric antral vascular ectasia ('watermelon stomach')

This is an uncommon condition that predominately affects middle aged and elderly women, causing either iron deficiency anaemia or a more brisk acute upper GI haemorrhage. Its colloquial name is derived from its endoscopic appearance, with red streaks radiating out from the pylorus of the stomach (Fig. 2).

Having excluded a colonic cause for anaemia, treatment can be with simple iron replacement therapy or the lesions may be treated endoscopically with either laser or argon beam photocoagulation. Hormone replacement therapy may be helpful, as may transexamic acid.

Angiodysplasia

With the widespread use of colonoscopy, this is increasingly recognised as a cause of iron deficiency anaemia affecting the middle aged and elderly. Small lesions occur, predominately in the caecum and right side of the colon, but they may occur throughout the length of the GI tract and usually cause chronic slow blood loss. The lesions appear as red blushes endoscopically and are due to fragile ectatic mucosal vessels (Fig. 3).

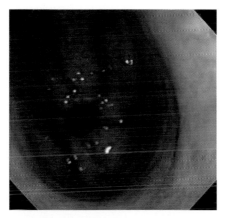

Fig. 2 **Watermelon stomach.**

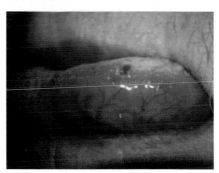

Fig. 3 **Oral telangiectases.**

If lesions are discovered incidentally and there has been no evidence of GI bleeding, then they can be left alone. If bleeding has occurred, then lesions can be treated by sclerotherapy or by ablation with either laser therapy or a heater probe. Certainty that the lesions were responsible for causing the anaemia is only possible when the anaemia does not recur. Right hemicolectomy may be necessary in intractable cases.

Hereditary haemorrhagic telangiectasia ('Osler–Weber–Rendu disease')

This is an autosomal dominant condition that may present in childhood with recurrent nosebleeds, but presents in later adult life with recurrent GI bleeding. Small raised vascular blebs occur under the tongue (Fig. 3) and around the lips as well as throughout the GI tract. Treatment of GI lesions is similar to that for angiodysplasia and includes endoscopic ablation, hormone replacement therapy and occasionally surgery.

Table 1 **Gastrointestinal causes of iron deficiency anaemia**

Upper GI causes
Gastric ulcers
Gastric erosions/gastritis
Oesophagitis
Gastric vascular antral ectasia
Angiodysplasia
Previous partial gastrectomy

Small bowel causes
Coeliac disease
Small bowel ulcers (NSAIDs)
Crohn's disease
Tumours
Hookworm

Large bowel causes
Neoplasia (polyps/cancers)
Angiodysplasia
Telangiectasia
Ulcerative colitis

Iron deficiency anaemia
- Anaemia should be confirmed to be due to iron deficiency by demonstrating a low serum ferritin.
- Unless it is due to menorrhagia, iron deficiency requires investigation.
- Always consider coeliac disease as a possible cause, in whatever age, and use anti-endomysial antibodies as a screening test.

LOWER GASTROINTESTINAL TRACT BLEEDING

Although a rather non-specific term, lower gastrointestinal (GI) bleeding is widely used to describe bleeding that occurs from the colon. It can usefully be divided into overt or occult bleeding. Overt or gross bleeding is remarkably common, with up to 15% of adults having reported red blood on the toilet paper following defaecation. The majority of these will be due to bleeding from haemorrhoids, which is dealt with on page 65. Brisk, more continuous colonic bleeding may be due to diverticular disease, or angiodysplasia (see p. 69), whilst colonic neoplasms most often present with occult GI bleeding. Other causes include colitis, colonic varices and intussusception of the colon, whilst Meckel's diverticulum is the most common cause of lower GI bleeding in children.

DIVERTICULAR BLEEDING

The vasa recta are branches of the marginal artery that supply the colon. They penetrate the muscular layer of the colon to supply the mucosa and it is at this point that diverticulae develop. Consequently, the penetrating vessels are only covered by mucosa and erosion at this site results in haemorrhage. Bleeding from diverticulae occurs in 3–5% of patients with diverticulae; it usually stops spontaneously but may occasionally require surgical resection. Diverticulae cause an acute bleed and are not a cause of chronic iron deficiency anaemia (see Fig 1. p. 40).

MECKEL'S DIVERTICULUM

This is a congenital anomaly of the gut which occurs in 3% of the population and arises within 3 feet (100 cm) of the ileo-caecal valve. Ulceration of acid-producing heterotopic gastric mucosa results in haemorrhage, but otherwise the condition often remains asymptomatic. A technetium-99m pertechnetate scan reveals ectopic gastric mucosa but the test has a 25% false-negative rate.

PNEUMATOSIS CYSTOIDES INTESTINALES

This is a rare condition in which patients may be symptomatic or have colitis-like symptoms. Air-filled cysts with a characteristic appearance occur in the colon (Fig. 1). The aetiology is unclear and the condition may be treated by oxygen therapy.

COLONIC POLYPS

The terminology applied to colonic polyps can be a little bewildering but is in fact quite simple; polyps may be described by their histological type including whether they are benign or malignant and by their morphology. Great interest has been aroused in adenomatous polyps because of their potential to become malignant, but a number of other polyps exist which have either no malignant potential or a low risk of becoming malignant.

All polyps may be described as sessile (lacking a stalk), pedunculated (with a stalk), or flat (Figs 2 and 3).

Hyperplastic or metaplastic polyps

Either term may be used and describes small, less than 5 mm, sessile polyps, which are more frequent in the distal colon and appear to get more common with age. Macroscopically indistinguishable from small adenomatous polyps, they are thought to carry no malignant potential and do not appear to be associated with adenomatous polyps elsewhere in the colon. Histologically, they reveal a well-differentiated epithelium but the crypts are elongated and the epithelial cells appear papillary. There is no cellular atypia and mitoses occur as normal in the base of the crypts. They are usually removed at endoscopy because they cannot be distinguished from small adenomas macroscopically, but if discovered at flexible sigmoidoscopy they are not an indication for full colonoscopy.

Inflammatory polyps or pseudopolyps

As the name suggests, these polyps are associated with chronic inflammation and represent the exuberant regeneration of mucosa following injury and ulceration. They may be small and multiple or may be singular and large and macroscopically indistinguishable from a large neoplastic polyp. They are often associated with ulcerative colitis and may form mucosal bridges across the lumen of the colon as they heal. They carry no malignant potential but histology has to confirm their inflammatory aetiology. Histology reveals inflammation and granulation tissue (Fig. 4).

Peutz–Jeghers polyps

Peutz–Jeghers syndrome is inherited as an autosomal dominant and is characterised by mucosal pigmentation and GI polyps. Polyps may occur throughout the length of the GI tract and have a characteristic histological appearance. Bands of muscle fibres rise from the muscularis mucosae and branch in a tree-like fashion

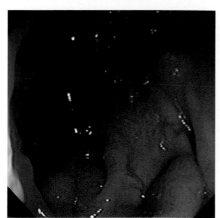

Fig. 1 **Pneumatosis coli.**

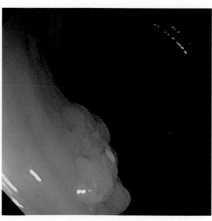

Fig. 2 **Sessile colonic polyp.**

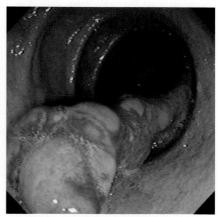

Fig. 3 **Pedunculated colonic polyp.**

to produce the polyp. Originally thought to have no malignant potential, they are now recognised as having a low risk of malignant change and should be removed. The polyps are often on a long stalk and may also induce intussusception, particularly when they occur in the small bowel. The syndrome is also associated with an increased risk of developing other tumours elsewhere, such as in the pancreas and ovary. The genetic defect has been located to the STK11 gene on chromosome 19.

Adenomatous polyps

A histological spectrum exists for adenomatous polyps, with the following range of types:

- tubular, in which more than 80% of the glands are branching
- tubulovillous
- villous, in which at least 80% of the glands are villiform, i.e. extend straight down from the surface of the polyp, creating villous-like projections to its surface.

The interest in adenomatous polyps has developed because it was recognised that colorectal cancers usually develop from pre-existing adenomatous polyps ('adenoma–carcinoma sequence'). This was demonstrated by following up patients who had previously been shown by barium enema to have a polypoid lesion. Over a 5-year period, 10% of these patients developed cancers at the site of the polyp. Also, it has been demonstrated that resection of all adenomatous polyps during endoscopy reduces the subsequent risk of colorectal cancer by up to 90%.

Size and histological type influence the chance of malignant change. Tubular adenomas, which are often small, have a low risk of malignant change; villous adenomas, which are often larger when discovered, have a higher risk of either being malignant at the time of discovery or of subsequently becoming malignant.

- Polyps below 1 cm in size have a low risk of malignant change and grow in a non-linear fashion; some may regress and disappear, whilst others may not grow at all.
- Polyps of > 1 cm on average take 5.5 years to undergo malignant transformation, demonstrating that the adenoma–carcinoma sequence is a slow process.
- Polyps of 1–2 cm often have a higher villous component and up to 10% may exhibit malignant change.
- Polyps larger than 2 cm have a 50% chance of being malignant.

Malignant polyps are those that following resection are shown to have areas of malignancy. They are deemed non-invasive when the malignant cells have not crossed the muscularis mucosae, as the lymphatic drainage does not extend up above this layer and therefore the chance of malignant dissemination is very low. Therefore endoscopic resection can usually be considered definitive treatment.

Management of adenomatous polyps
There is considerable debate as to the most appropriate way to follow up patients who have been shown to have a colonic polyp. However, the recommendations in Figure 5 would be widely accepted.

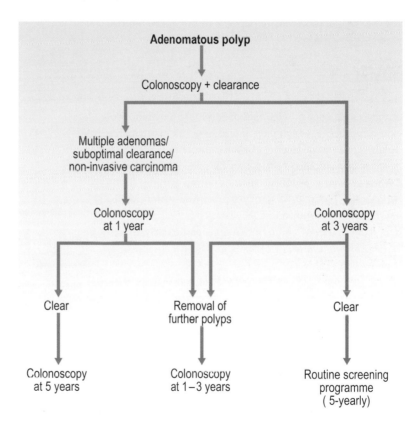

Fig. 5 **Follow-up of adenomatous polyps.**

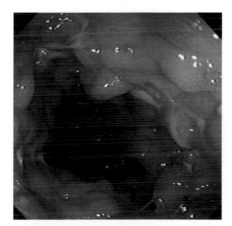

Fig. 4 **Inflammatory pseudopolyps.**

Lower gastrointestinal tract bleeding
- Lower GI bleeding usually stops spontaneously.
- All lower GI bleeding requires investigation.
- Adenomatous polyps have the potential to grow and undergo malignant change, with tubular adenomas having the lowest risk, and villous adenomas the highest.
- Adenomatous polyps should be completely excised and the patients entered into a surveillance programme.
- Hyperplastic/metaplastic polyps and inflammatory polyps have no risk of malignant change; Peutz–Jeghers polyps have a low risk of neoplastic transformation.

COLORECTAL CANCER I

EPIDEMIOLOGY

About 6% of the population living to the age of 80 in the USA will develop colo-rectal cancer (CRC). 90% develop from pre-existing adenomas, 75% of the total will be sporadic with no family history, and 1% will develop in patients with ulcerative colitis. Colonic cancer has an equal age/sex distribution, but rectal carcinoma is more common in men. The mean age of presentation of sporadic CRC is 67 years (90% develop after the age of 50) but it is lower in familial CRC.

There is a wide geographic variation, with rates up to 20 times higher in the Western world, but countries with a previously low incidence are showing rises, such as Japan where there has been a 40% increase over the last 30 years. The incidence of CRC in migrants also rapidly assumes that in the local population, becoming almost equal within a generation.

The distribution of CRC within the colon is also changing, with a rise in the incidence of right-sided tumours (Fig. 1), which means that at least 40% of tumours would not be reached by flexible sigmoidoscopy.

AETIOLOGY

Diet

An increased incidence of CRC is recognised with a number of dietary factors such as a high meat intake, low calcium, vitamin D or folate intake, high alochol consumption (especially rectal cancer in men), smoking, increased fat intake and obesity. Meat, when cooked at > 200°C, such as during grilling, frying and barbecuing, produces heterocyclic amines, which in fast acetylators have been linked to CRC development. Factors that appear to reduce risk are a high fibre intake, particularly as vegetables, and use of aspirin or other NSAIDs, which appear to confer protection (Table 1).

The role of fibre has been recognised since the early 1970s when low CRC rates amongst Africans were attributed to their high fibre intake. However, dietary fibre is non-digested plant material and contains starches and non-starch polysaccharides, so the exact protective component is unclear. Although the

mechanism is unclear, the protection given by vegetables may be due to micronutrients and antioxidants, as well as increased stool bulk and decreased transit time, resulting in less exposure of the colon to carcinogens. Also, the production of the short-chain fatty acid, butyrate, which is derived from fibre, may also be protective. It is a colonocyte nutrient that has effects on cellular proliferation and differentiation.

Genetic factors

A number of inherited syndromes have been recognised and, in some, the genetic abnormalities have been identified (Table 2). However, even in sporadic cases, which form the bulk of CRCs,

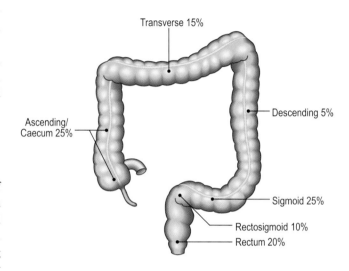

Fig. 1 **Sites of colorectal cancer.**

Table 1 **Factors that affect the risk of developing colorectal cancer**

Increase risk	Lower risk
Red meat consumption (left colon)	Vegetable consumption
Well-cooked meat	Folate intake
Alcohol	Selenium
Eggs	NSAID/aspirin use
High body mass index	High calcium intake
Smoking	
Previous cholecystectomy (right colon)	

Table 2 **Hereditary cancer syndromes**

Syndrome	GI manifestations	Other clinical features	Genetics
Hereditary non-polyposis colon cancer (HNPCC)	Small numbers of colorectal polyps	Muir – Torre variant – with sebaceous adenomas, basal cell epitheliomas	Autosomal dominant Mutations: MLH1 (chromosome 3p) MLH2 (2p) MSH6 (2p) PMS 1 (2q) PMS 2 (7q)
Hereditary polyposis syndromes Familial adenomatous polyposis (FAP)/Gardner's syndrome	100–1000s of adenomas in colon, stomach and small bowel	Osteomas, desmoid tumours, epidermoid cysts, congenital hypertrophy of retinal pigmented epithelium	Autosomal dominant APC gene (5q)
Turcot syndrome	Colorectal polyps	Brain tumours	Autosomal dominant APC gene/MLH1
Peutz–Jeghers syndrome	Hamartomas throughout gut	Pigmented skin lesions	Autosomal dominant STK11 gene (19p)
Cowden disease	Hamartomatous polyps in colon and stomach	Thyroid adenomas/cancers Breast cancer in women	Autosomal dominant PTEN gene (10q)
Familial juvenile polyposis	Juvenile polyps in colon/GIT	Malrotation. Hydrocephalus	Autosomal dominant (in some families)

a familial component is well recognised as risk increases with increasing numbers of affected relatives (Table 3).

Hereditary colon cancer can develop in colons where hundreds of polyps have developed (the hereditary polyposis syndromes), or in families where there is an inherited predisposition to form small numbers of polyps that later become malignant (hereditary non-polyposis colon cancer – HNPCC). Table 4 defines HNPCC.

In familial adenomatous polyposis (FAP), which is inherited as an autosomal dominant, the genetic abnormality has been termed the adenomatous polyposis coli (APC) gene and is located on the long arm of chromosome 5 (5q21). Somatic mutations also occur at this site in sporadic cases of CRC.

HNPCC is also inherited in an autosomal dominant fashion and several genetic defects have now been identified. Genes termed MLH, MSH and PMS are involved in repairing DNA during replication, and abnormalities in them lead to replication errors. These genes have been located on chromosomes 2, 3 and 7. Somatic mutations at these points have also been recognised in some sporadic cases of CRC.

Oncogenes normally play a part in regulation of cell growth but mutations are commonly recognised in CRC such that altered cellular proliferation can occur, predisposing to adenoma formation. K-ras is one such oncogene which frequently undergoes mutation during the development of colonic adenomas.

CLINICAL FEATURES

CRC can present in a number of different ways dependent largely on their site. Right-sided CRC usually presents with features of anaemia, and so can present late. Visible rectal bleeding is more commonly associated with left-sided lesions, and is usually seen as blood mixed in with the stool. The combination of rectal bleeding and a change in bowel habit is the symptom complex with the highest association with CRC and always requires investigation. Abdominal pain is often non-specific and the vast majority of patients with pain do not have CRC. Tenesmus can occur with rectal lesions. Large bowel obstruction is also a common presentation but often patients will have had other symptoms preceding presentation. Abdominal examination is often normal although a mass or enlarged liver may be felt in advanced disease. Rectal masses can be detected by digital examination of the anorectal canal.

Rigid sigmoidoscopy of the unprepared bowel is widely practised but the view is often poor owing to faeces. Flexible sigmoidoscopy following an enema gives a more extensive, better quality view. Sub-sequent barium enema examination or colonoscopy is required for visualization of the right colon (Fig. 2).

In FAP, individuals develop 100s or 1000s of colonic polyps during the second and third decade, with colonic cancer developing by the age of 40. Screening in affected families begins in the second and third decades, and if more than 100 adenomas are identified, this is confirmation of inheritance and colectomy is required. Gardner's syndrome has been traced to the same APC gene as FAP, and is probably a variant of FAP. There are multiple colonic adenomas, with osteomas, retinal pigment epithelium abnormalities and upper GI polyps.

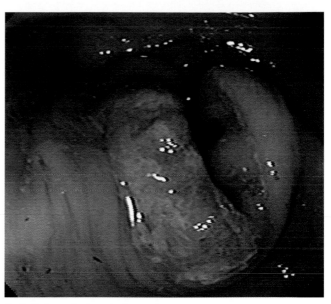

Fig. 2 **Endoscopic view of colo-rectal cancer.**

Table 3 **Family history and estimated lifetime risk of developing colorectal cancer**

Number of affected individuals	Attributed lifetime risk
No affected relatives	1 : 50
1 first-degree relative	1 : 17
1 first- and 1 second-degree relative	1 : 12
1 first-degree relative age < 45	1 : 10
Both parents affected	1 : 8.5
2 first-degree relatives (not both parents)	1 : 6
3 first-degree relatives	1 : 2

Three affected first-degree relatives suggests a dominant inheritance.
First-degree relative = parent, sibling; second-degree relative = uncle/aunt, grandparent

Table 4 **Definition of hereditary non-polyposis colorectal cancer (HNPCC)**

- At least three relatives with CRC (at least one must be a first-degree relative of the other two)
- CRC involving at least two generations
- One or more CRCs before age 50
- If HNPCC is limited to the colon it is termed site-specific HNPCC, HNPCC type a, or Lynch syndrome I
- If family members are also prone to developing cancers of the female genital tract, it is termed HNPCC type b, Lynch syndrome II, or cancer family syndrome

Colorectal cancer I

- Individuals with no family history have a 1 : 50 risk of developing CRC, which rises to 1 : 17 with one affected first-degree relative.
- Because of the adenoma–carcinoma sequence, CRC has the potential for effective screening prior to the development of cancer.
- Early detection and treatment of CRC improves survival.
- Familial predisposition to CRC may occur with either polyposis syndromes (development of multiple colonic adenomas) or non-polyposis syndromes where few adenomas develop.
- Change in bowel habit with blood in the stool are the symptoms most closely associated with CRC.

COLORECTAL CANCER II

SCREENING

Huge interest in the possibility of screening for CRC has developed as doctors and politicians try to establish which modality is most practically and financially acceptable. CRC fulfils a number of criteria essential for an effective screening programme. It represents a significant public health problem, the natural history is amenable to early premalignant detection and treatment, there are safe, sensitive, specific screening techniques and screening may be cost-effective. As yet, there is not a national screening programme in the UK but this seems to be imminent. Choosing how to screen people is more problematic as a balance between cost, sensitivity of the test and patient acceptability has to be achieved. Because of its rapidity and lack of requirement for extensive bowel preparation, flexible sigmoidoscopy, which will only detect left-sided lesions, appears to be in the forefront as a screening modality, particularly if coupled with faecal occult blood testing, which will help detect right-sided lesions (Fig. 1). Deciding upon a suitable age to screen people is a balance between screening too early when lesions may not have

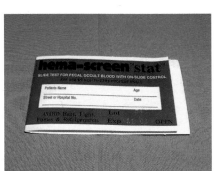

Fig. 1 **FOB testing.**

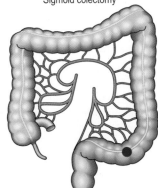

Fig. 2 **Barium enema of colon cancer.**

Right hemicolectomy

Extended right hemicolectomy

Transverse colectomy

Left hemicolectomy

Sigmoid colectomy

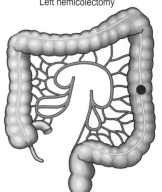

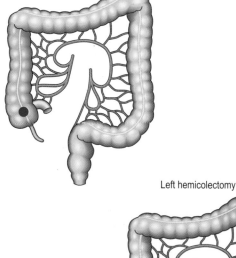

Fig. 3 **Resections for colonic cancer.**

developed and screening too late when cancers have formed. A screening programme would have massive implications for endoscopists, not only because of the requirements of flexible sigmoidoscopy but also for subsequent colonoscopy when lesions were detected, and also for surgical resources for patients where tumours were detected.

INVESTIGATIONS

Patients requiring lower GI investigation at presentation normally undergo a sigmoidoscopy and barium enema (Fig. 2) (the sigmoidoscopy performed because rectal lesions are often not well visualised at barium enema), or colonoscopy. Colonoscopy is more sensitive and can detect lesions smaller than 1 cm, which barium enema is usually unable to do, and also allows biopsy and polyp removal. However, compared to barium enema, colonoscopy is more time-consuming, less comfortable for the patient, requires analgesia and sedation and has a higher risk of procedure-related morbidity. Large lesions are usually readily detected but there still remains the problem of missing small lesions. Following detection of a tumour, the rest of the colon requires visualisation, if not already performed, as 5% of patients have synchronous tumours elsewhere in the colon.

STAGING

Various staging methods are used but most are modifications of Dukes' description in the 1930s, which has prognostic implications following treatment (Table 1). The TNM classification is also widely used (see p. 28).

TREATMENT

Surgery aims to excise the lesion with at least a 5-cm clearance, plus the entire mesentery, including the blood vessels that supply the tumour (Fig. 3). If rectal lesions are high enough and a 2-cm margin of clearance above the anal canal is possible, then an anterior resection (via the abdomen) is possible. Low lesions require an abdominoperineal resection where the distal sigmoid, rectum and anus are all removed via abdominal and perineal incisions and a permanent sigmoid colostomy is fashioned. Rectal lesions can also be dealt with via the rec-

tum using transanal microsurgical techniques, allowing mucosal resection.

Advanced tumours causing obstructive symptoms often occur in patients who are unfit for surgery or in whom there are distant metastases. In these cases, flexible metal stents can be placed endoscopically, which can offer good palliation (Fig. 4). Tumours can also be treated with laser therapy in an attempt to maintain colonic patency.

Adjuvant chemotherapy, particularly using 5-fluorouracil (5-FU), offers some palliative advantage, and other chemotherapy combinations are being trialled. Preoperative radiotherapy to rectal lesions has been shown to confer benefit.

Solitary liver metastases are now being more aggressively treated, either with local resection or with cryotherapy. Chemotherapy is also being targeted by the placement of portal catheters, through which the chemotherapy is given.

Following resection, follow-up to detect local or distant recurrence is often undertaken, although this probably does not affect long-term survival because local recurrence is difficult to treat and is often accompanied by more distant

spread. However, it should not be forgotten that these patients are at increased risk of developing further CRCs and should be entered into a screening programme for this.

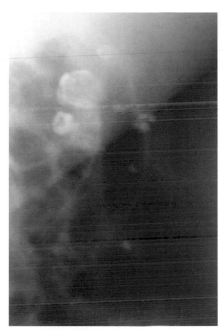

Fig. 4 **Colonic stent.**

Table 1 **Dukes' staging for colorectal cancer (with subsequent modification)**

Stage	Extent	Approximate survival rates
Dukes' A	Limited to bowel wall	80% 5-year survival
Dukes' B	Through bowel wall	55% 5-year survival
Dukes' C1	1–4 local lymph nodes affected	45% 5-year survival
Dukes' C2	> 4 regional nodes	15% 5-year survival
Dukes' D	Distant metastases	1% 5-year survival

Colorectal cancer II

- Individuals with no family history have a 1:50 risk of developing CRC, which rises to 1:17 with one affected first-degree relative.
- Because of the adenoma–carcinoma sequence, CRC has the potential for effective screening prior to the development of cancer.
- Early detection and treatment of CRC improves survival.
- Familial predisposition to CRC may occur with either polyposis syndromes (development of multiple colonic adenomas) or non-polyposis syndromes where few adenomas develop.
- Change in bowel habit with blood in the stool are the symptoms most closely associated with CRC.

THE CLINICAL APPROACH

HISTORY

The inquisitorial skills of the physician are most required when taking a history from a jaundiced patient or one with liver disease. Aspects of the recent, middle and distant past can all be relevant in these patients and probing and reminding patients of things that they may have forgotten or felt unimportant is necessary. It also brings great pleasure to the physician when finally the critical piece of information to make a diagnosis is elicited.

When interrogating a patient with a recent onset of jaundice, it is usual to establish whether the jaundice is cholestatic/obstructive or of another cause. Pale stools, dark urine and itch are the cardinal features of this type of jaundice and patients usually acknowledge these features enthusiastically when prompted. Preceding episodic right upper quadrant pain, rigors and a family history of gallstones point to common bile duct (CBD) stones as a cause for the jaundice, whereas an absence of pain associated with weight loss is more suggestive of a malignant cause such as carcinoma of the head of the pancreas. A thorough drug history is essential and sometimes difficult as this should include prescribed and over-the-counter preparations taken for up to 6 months beforehand. A variety of drugs are recognised as causes of a cholestatic jaundice (see p. 100). Previous visits or residence overseas should be documented.

Patients who develop jaundice as a result of a hepatitic process may have a period of cholestasis in the early phases of the illness, but this feature is not usually prominent, whereas a feeling of malaise or systemic upset is more common. Enquiry should again include a drug history (including recreational drugs), contact history of other individuals with jaundice, foreign travel, sexual contact, family history and past medical history including previous blood transfusion. Deception by patients is not unheard of, particularly when talking about previous recreational drug usage, sexual contact, alcohol usage and deliberate self-harm due to drug overdosage. In the setting of an unexplained acute hepatitis, paracetamol overdose should always be considered.

Taking an accurate alcohol history requires tact and a non-judgmental approach if accurate values are to be obtained. This part of the history should be elicited from all patients, including those without GI disease, as alcohol can affect many systems, both singly and in combination.

Previous medical and surgical history is essential particularly if there has been hepatobiliary surgery. The family history may be revealing in diseases that are inherited or have a genetic component. Men with haemochromatosis may describe their father having died at a relatively young age with 'liver cancer' and a brother with 'liver problems'. The firm diagnosis of haemochromatosis and hepatocellular cancer complicating this condition may never have been made, but may be the case. Women with an autoimmune hepatitis are more likely to have relatives with a history of other autoimmune diseases.

Exposure during employment, with particular reference to solvents, may also be revealing.

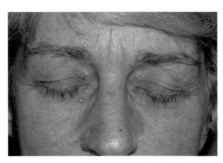

Fig. 1 **Xanthelasma in woman with primary biliary cirrhosis.**

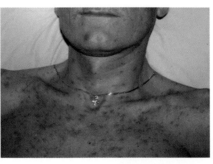

Fig. 2 **Spider naevi on chest wall.**

EXAMINATION

Occasionally, the pigmentation associated with haemochromatosis, or spider naevi is visible on general inspection. The hands may show palmar erythema ('liver palms'), finger clubbing, leuconychia (pallor of the nail bed associated with hypoalbuminaemia), Dupuytren's contracture (tethering of the palmar fascia) and a slow flap of hepatic encephalopathy.

Jaundice is best seen in the white of the sclera, where the distinction between the greenish discoloration of chronic jaundice due to obstruction and the yellow tinge caused by haemolysis can be made. Xanthelasma may also be seen on the eyelids (Fig. 1). Spider naevi are visible over the arms and upper chest (Fig.2), and gynaecomastia may be seen in males. Abdominal distension may be due to fat, ascites, or gas, and percussion with shifting dullness will help distinguish ascites (Fig. 3). Rarely, veins are visible radiating from the umbilicus (caput medusae); these occur in portal hypertension.

Hepatomegaly should be identified and the consistency and surface of the organ felt; a hard irregular liver has a characteristic feel and denotes a liver with metastatic disease – once felt it is not forgotten. The liver may feel firm and smooth in cirrhosis, where the presence of splenomegaly suggests portal hypertension.

Small testicles are seen with gynaecomastia as a feature of feminisation in chronic liver disease.

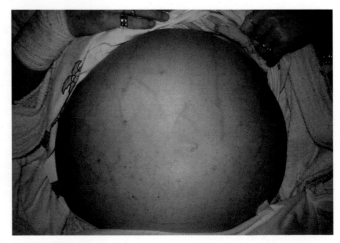

Fig. 3 **Gross ascites.**

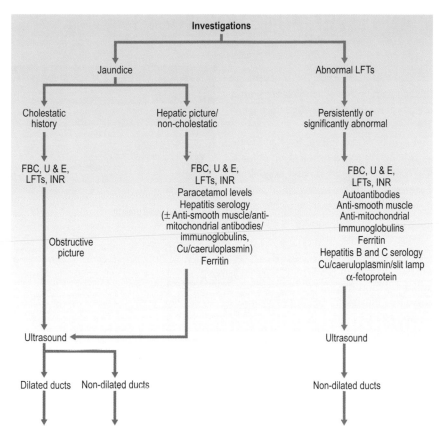

Fig. 4 **Investigation algorithm for jaundice and abnormal liver function tests.**

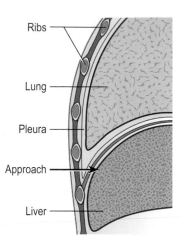

Fig. 5 **Positioning of liver biopsy.**

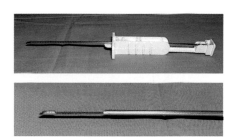

Fig. 6 **Trucut liver biopsy needle.**

INVESTIGATIONS

The investigation algorithm (Fig. 4) is a guide to how patients can be investigated to get to the diagnosis with least resource wastage. However, atypical presentations occur and flexibility in approach is essential.

Liver biopsy

This is a widely performed procedure in gastroenterology, and clinicians must be aware of the potential hazards and the associated mortality, so that informed consent from the patient can be obtained (Table 1). The procedure may be performed under ultrasound guidance or 'blindly' following percussion. Percutaneous biopsy should not be performed in the presence of bile duct obstruction, ascites, skin sepsis or abnormal clotting. Ultrasound guidance is most useful if a solitary lesion requires biopsy.

Following consent, blood is drawn for an FBC with platelet count, clotting studies and grouping and saving, to allow rapid cross-match in the event of haemorrhage. The risk of haemorrhage rises with lower platelet counts and rising prothrombin times, and percutaneous biopsy should not be performed if the platelet count is < 60 000/mm³ and the international normalised ratio (INR) is > 1.4. In these circumstances a transjugular approach is necessary.

The upper border of the liver is identified by percussion (dull) and is marked, on both inspiration and expiration, in the mid-axillary line. The area is cleaned and then infiltrated with local anaesthetic down to the liver capsule. The needle is advanced whilst the patient is in expiration so that the lung is as small as possible and the liver in its highest position, allowing penetration of the needle through the potential space of the lower pleural reflection (Fig. 5). Confirmation of liver penetration is made by observing oscillation of the syringe and needle during gentle respiration (this does not occur if the lung has been penetrated). A small incision is made with a blade and, using the same technique of advancing during expiration, the biopsy needle is advanced and the biopsy taken. Various biopsy needles are produced, such as the modified Menghini and Trucut types (Fig. 6).

If clotting abnormalities preclude percutaneous liver biopsy, a biopsy can be obtained via the jugular and hepatic veins – the transjugular route. Any bleeding that occurs tends to be into the hepatic vein, rather than intra-abdominally.

Table 1 **Potential complications following liver biopsy**

- Internal haemorrhage
- Bile leakage
- Pneumothorax
- Haemoptysis
- Gallbladder perforation
- Inadvertent renal biopsy

The clinical approach

- Detailed history must determine the type of jaundice (obstructive/hepatitic/haemolytic), include contacts, travel, drug usage (prescribed and recreational), blood transfusion history, family history and past medical and surgical history.
- Examination should demonstrate features of chronic liver disease if present.
- Investigations should exclude haemolysis, then establish whether the hepatobiliary system is obstructed (usually best done with ultrasound).
- An obstructed system will usually require ERCP for both diagnosis and treatment.
- Liver biopsy should be considered if the diagnosis is in doubt, or for staging purposes. It is a potentially risky procedure which should only be performed when necessary.

BILIRUBIN METABOLISM AND LIVER FUNCTION TESTS

BILIRUBIN METABOLISM

It is useful to have a working knowledge of bilirubin metabolism when dealing with a jaundiced patient (Fig. 1) not only to help one understand the mechanisms by which jaundice may have developed but also to help interpret the liver tests.

Bilirubin is produced in the reticuloendothelial system of the spleen, liver and bone marrow predominantly from haem degradation, although cytochromes and myoglobin contribute a small amount (Fig. 2). Unconjugated bilirubin is tightly bound to albumin and is actively taken up by the hepatocyte. Renal excretion of unconjugated bilirubin does not occur owing to its tight binding to albumin. Following cleavage from albumin, the bilirubin is conjugated with glucuronide, using the enzyme UDP-glucuronyl transferase, in the endoplasmic reticulum of the hepatocyte. Conjugated bilirubin is water soluble and is actively excreted across the canalicular membrane into the bile canaliculus using an ATP-dependent pump. The majority is then excreted into the stool, but some deconjugation occurs in the bowel and a small amount of this urobilinogen is reabsorbed and then excreted in the urine.

The commonest causes of jaundice involve a defect in metabolism of bilirubin or its excretion. However, increased turnover of red cells, as in haemolysis, may saturate the system responsible for the disposal of bilirubin and result in jaundice.

Conjugated bilirubin gives a direct reaction with the Van der Berg test and is confusingly termed direct bilirubin, whilst the protein bound to unconjugated bilirubin has to be precipitated prior to assay and is termed indirect bilirubin.

LIVER FUNCTION TESTS

Strictly, most of the tests that are referred to as 'liver function tests' (LFTs) are not tests of liver function but rather assays that give information about hepatocyte damage, enzyme induction or cholestasis. Of the commonly performed tests, only those for prothrombin time and level of serum albumin might be termed tests of function. It is essential to know the source of the various enzymes measured in order for them to help in diagnosis.

Aminotransferases

Alanine aminotransferase (ALT) is a cytosolic (i.e. intracellular) enzyme of hepatocytes and is liberated into the circulation following hepatocellular damage. It is relatively liver specific, unlike aspartate aminotransferase (AST), which also occurs in cardiac muscle, striated muscle, kidney, brain and red blood cells. Slight elevations (two to five times the normal range < 250 IU) occur commonly in many liver conditions, whilst marked elevations (20–40 times, or values > 1000 IU) tend to occur with a hepatitis, whether viral or drug induced.

Usually the AST/ALT ratio is 1, but in alcoholic liver disease the ratio is often greater than 2.

Gamma glutamyl transpeptidase (GGT)

This is an inducible microsomal enzyme, which may rise, to a variable extent, in many liver conditions. It does not signify damage, merely that its production has been induced. Regular alcohol consumption may induce it, but it is a poor marker of alcohol abuse as values may be normal in alcohol abusers. It can be used to monitor abstinence in those in whom alcohol has caused a rise. Drugs, such as anticonvulsants, oestrogens, and warfarin commonly induce the enzyme and lead to a rise in the serum concen-

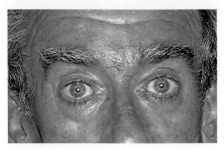

Fig. 1 **Jaundiced patient.**

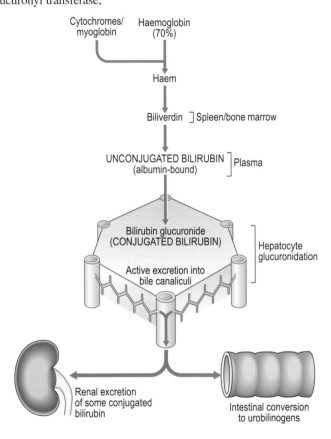

Fig. 2 **Bilirubin metabolism.**

tration. It is found in various extrahepatic tissues such as kidney, heart and lung, but not in bone, and can be used to help determine whether alkaline phosphatase is of bony or hepatic origin. An elevated GGT with a raised alkaline phosphatase implies hepatic origin of the AP.

Patients are occasionally referred for investigation of an isolated elevated GGT. This is usually unnecessary – either a drug or alcohol may be responsible, but even if there is no ready explanation further investigation is not warranted.

Alkaline phosphatase (AP)

Various isoenzymes of AP exist denoting mainly hepatic or bony origin but AP is also found in small bowel, kidney and placenta. AP from the liver is produced in the canalicular membrane and also the bile duct epithelium. Following obstruction of the biliary tree, AP production is induced, which leads to a rise in the serum concentration. In cholestasis (where there is no mechanical obstruction) bile acids may facilitate the release of AP. Discrimination between hepatic and bony AP can be made by specific assay of isoenzymes, or it can be assumed that the AP is of bony origin if the GGT is normal.

The AP often rises modestly in many liver diseases, but is most markedly elevated in ductal obstruction, cholestasis and infiltration of the liver by tumour. There may also be modest rises in hypermetabolic states such as thyrotoxicosis and pyrexial illnesses of any cause.

The half-life of AP is about 7 days, so relief of extrahepatic obstruction may take a few days to result in a fall in the serum AP.

Synthetic function of the liver

Albumin

Albumin is only synthesised in the liver and about 10 g is made each day. Under normal conditions the half-life is 20 days, but very many extrahepatic conditions influence the serum concentration. The serum albumin concentration is affected by nutritional status, general metabolic state and urinary and faecal losses. It is therefore a poor marker of hepatic function.

Clotting factors (prothrombin time)

All the clotting factors except factor VIII are made within the liver. The vitamin K-dependent factors (II, VII, IX and X) may be inadequately produced in malabsorption of vitamin K owing to obstructive jaundice or cholestasis, but are rapidly synthesised when parenteral vitamin K is given. Factor VII has the shortest half-life of these factors of 6 hours and can be used to monitor patients with acute liver failure.

The prothrombin time reflects a number of clotting factors of the extrinsic clotting pathway but may be prolonged for reasons other than impaired liver synthesis. These include vitamin K malabsorption, warfarin administration and disseminated intravascular coagulation. A prolongation of the prothrombin time because of liver disease, as opposed to obstruction, will not completely correct with parenteral vitamin K administration, and thus reflects liver function. Measurement of prothrombin time may be particularly helpful in patients with acute liver disease such as that following a paracetamol overdose, when changes in the prothrombin time over the first few hours after the overdose have prognostic implications.

α-fetoprotein

This is the fetal equivalent of albumin, which largely replaces it by the end of the first year of life. It is produced during times of hepatic regeneration, leading to a modest rise in serum concentrations but rises substantially with hepatocellular carcinoma, for which it is used as a marker.

Ferritin

This major intracellular iron storage protein is used as a marker for haemochromatosis when elevated levels are observed. However, it is also an acute phase protein and rises with many liver complaints. Care has to be taken in interpreting an elevated value before making a diagnosis of haemochromatosis.

PATTERNS OF ABNORMAL LFTs

Once armed with the specific details of liver tests, clinicians have to recognise the common patterns that occur, leading them to appropriate investigation and making a diagnosis. This is similar to interpreting ECGs. The patterns that are seen include cholestasis or obstruction, hepatitis, mild hepatocellular changes and non-specific rises in the enzymes (Table 1).

The gastroenterologist will also often be asked to interpret or investigate a number of patterns of LFTs which are less commonly seen by the generalist and which may or may not require investigation (Table 2).

Table 1 **Commonly seen patterns of LFTs**

	Obstruction/ cholestasis	Hepatitis	Mild hepatocellular damage	Gilbert's syndrome/ haemolysis
Bilirubin	+++	++	+	+ (indirect)
ALT	+	++++	+	N
AP	+++	+	+	N
GGT	++	++	+	N

ALT = alanine aminotransferase; AP = alkaline phosphatase; GGT = gamma glutamyl transpeptidase; N = normal

Table 2 **Causes of some commonly seen LFT abnormalities**

Abnormality	Cause
Marked aminotransferase elevation (1000–2000 IU/l)	Viral hepatitis (e.g. hepatitis A) Drug-induced hepatitis (e.g. paracetamol) Shock liver (following hypotension)
Moderate persistent aminotransferase elevation (100–250 IU/l)	Chronic virus infection (e.g. hepatitis C) Ongoing alcohol abuse Medication (NSAIDs, statins) Immune hepatitis
Mild persistent aminotransferase elevation (50–100 IU/l)	As for moderate elevation Steatosis (obesity, diabetes mellitus, drugs)
Isolated elevated GGT (50–250 IU/l)	Alcohol Medication (OCP, anticonvulsants, warfarin) Steatosis (obesity)
Markedly raised AP, bilirubin and GGT (AP > 500 IU/l) Bilirubin > 50 μmol/l GGT > 200 IU/l	Obstruction (CBD stones, pancreatic cancer) Cholestasis (drugs, PBC, PSC) Infiltration by tumour (primary/secondary)

OCP = over-the-counter preparations; CBD = common bile duct; PBC = primary biliary cirrhosis, PSC = primary sclerosing cholangitis

Liver function tests

- Aminotransferases reflect hepatocellular damage; GGT is an inducible enzyme which does not reflect cellular damage; alkaline phosphatase rises most markedly in biliary obstruction, cholestasis and infiltration of the liver.
- Clotting studies are a useful method of monitoring progress in acute hepatitis, and they are one of the factors used to determine whether a patient with acute liver injury requires referral to a specialist liver unit.
- Albumin, and the clotting factors reflect true 'functional' tests, but the serum albumin concentration is affected by factors other than just hepatic synthesis.

ALCOHOLIC LIVER DISEASE I

BACKGROUND

Alcoholic beverages have been brewed and consumed since Egyptian times but it was recognised by the Greeks that excessive consumption could cause liver disease. Although the focus here is on the damage to the liver that may be caused by alcohol, it must be remembered that alcohol can cause profound social and personal damage as well as having wide-ranging physical effects. The World Health Organization estimates that 8% of Europeans and North Americans are excessive drinkers and that there may be as much as £2 billion lost to British industry per year owing to the effects of alcohol, and in the United States more than 20 times this amount.

The effects of alcohol can be seen in many organ systems and these may occur individually or in combination (Fig. 1).

However, it must not be forgotten that alcohol is also safely enjoyed by huge numbers around the world, and that there are potential health benefits to be accrued from its consumption, such as a reduction in ischaemic heart disease.

QUANTIFICATION AND SUSCEPTIBILITY

Quantifying the amount of alcohol a patient consumes is notoriously difficult as accuracy depends on patients' recall. It is said that women tend to underestimate their consumption whilst men exaggerate theirs. Either way, the most useful estimate will be achieved when trust is developed with the physician and a non-censorious approach is used. It is inadequate simply to record that a patient is a 'social' drinker, and the concept of a 'unit' of alcohol has been developed in

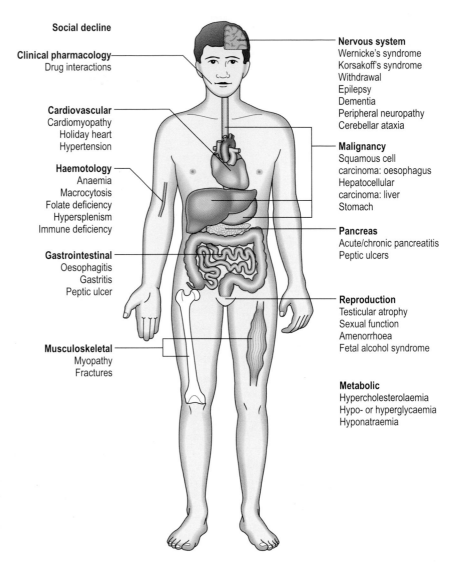

Fig. 1 **Effects of alcohol abuse.**

Social decline

Clinical pharmacology
Drug interactions

Cardiovascular
Cardiomyopathy
Holiday heart
Hypertension

Haemotology
Anaemia
Macrocytosis
Folate deficiency
Hypersplenism
Immune deficiency

Gastrointestinal
Oesophagitis
Gastritis
Peptic ulcer

Musculoskeletal
Myopathy
Fractures

Nervous system
Wernicke's syndrome
Korsakoff's syndrome
Withdrawal
Epilepsy
Dementia
Peripheral neuropathy
Cerebellar ataxia

Malignancy
Squamous cell
carcinoma: oesophagus
Hepatocellular
carcinoma: liver
Stomach

Pancreas
Acute/chronic pancreatitis
Peptic ulcers

Reproduction
Testicular atrophy
Sexual function
Amenorrhoea
Fetal alcohol syndrome

Metabolic
Hypercholesterolaemia
Hypo- or hyperglycaemia
Hyponatraemia

an attempt to make quantification more straightforward. This has the benefit of being simple to understand and the majority of patients are aware that a unit loosely represents one measure of spirit, a half pint of beer or a small glass of wine. The drawback is that beers vary widely in strength, as do wines, and home measures are usually highly variable. It is necessary to memorise some useful values and these are outlined in (Table 1).

Assessing whether a patient is abusing alcohol or alcohol-dependent may be aided by the 'CAGE' questionnaire, which relies on four questions that help identify this group (Table 2).

The British Government has published safe drinking recommendations (men < 28 units per week, women < 21

Table 1 Contents of alcoholic beverages

1 unit = 7.7 g alcohol
Grams of alcohol = Volume (ml) × Concentration (%) × 0.00798

Beers and lagers
Beer – bitter – 3.8% = 1.7 U in a 440-ml can = 13 g alcohol
Strong lager – 5.2% = 2.3 U in a 440-ml can = 18 g alcohol
Premium strength lager – 9.0% = 4.7 U in a 440-ml can = 36 g alcohol

Wine
Wine ~ 13% = 10 U in a conventional 750-ml bottle = 78 g alcohol
5 glasses/bottle (150 ml) = 2 U/glass

Spirits
Spirit ~ 40% = 29 U per 750-ml bottle = 223 g alcohol

Table 2 The 'CAGE' questionnaire

1 Have you ever felt that you should **Cut** down your drinking?
2 Have people **Annoyed** you by criticising your drinking?
3 Have you ever felt **Guilty** about your drinking?
4 Have you ever had an **Eye-opener** – an early morning drink to steady your nerves or help a hangover?
Three or four positive answers suggests a high probability of alcohol abuse or dependency

Table 3 **Patterns of blood test results pointing to alcohol abuse**

Test	Possible observed result
Full blood count	
Haemoglobin	Low, owing to GI bleed, marrow suppression
Platelets	Low, owing to marrow suppression, hypersplenism
MCV	Raised, owing to alcohol effect on bone marrow
Urea and electrolytes	
Sodium	Low, owing to total body water excess
Potassium	Low, owing to poor protein intake
Urea	Low, owing to decreased protein catabolism
	Raised, in the presence of GI bleed, hepatorenal syndrome
Creatinine	Raised, in the presence of hepatorenal syndrome
Liver tests	
Bilirubin	Raised, in the presence of significant liver disease
Aminotransferases (ALT, AST)	Raised, owing to hepatocellular disease, but can be almost normal, particularly in advanced disease
Alkaline phosphatase	Raised, when cholestasis present
GGT	Commonly raised, but can be elevated for very many other reasons, or may be normal
Others	
Vitamin B_{12}	Raised, liberated from damaged hepatocytes
Folic acid	Low, owing to malnourishment
Albumin	Low, owing to malnourishment, depressed hepatic synthesis
Prothrombin time	Prolonged, owing to depressed synthetic function of the liver
IgA	Raised
Blood alcohol	Raised, can be useful in patients who claim abstinence

units per week). This is a useful exercise as far as population education goes and, indeed, there is probably no risk of developing alcohol-related liver disease below these levels, but susceptibility to developing liver disease is highly variable and difficult to predict accurately for any one individual. Only 20% of heavy consumers of alcohol go on to develop liver disease, and perhaps just 5% develop cirrhosis. That is not to say that other organs will not be affected or that social and domestic interactions will not deteriorate at these consumption levels.

Not only the quantity, but also the pattern of drinking appears to be important, in that individuals who just drink one type of beverage at meal times are less likely to develop liver disease than those who mix drinks and consume alcohol away from meals. Co-existent diseases such as haemochromatosis or chronic viral hepatitis undoubtedly exacerbate the effects of alcohol on the liver.

There is probably a genetic component to the susceptibility to developing alcoholism, that is the addiction to alcohol, and also to the individual's response to alcohol. There is an increased risk of developing alcoholism in children of alcoholic parents. Various isoenzymes exist of the major enzymes responsible for metabolism of alcohol (Fig. 2). They have different rates of production or oxygenation of acetaldehyde, which is one of the potential injurious agents in the development of liver disease. Individuals who produce acetaldehyde rapidly, or metabolise it slowly may be those who are more likely to develop liver disease. Some alcohol dehydrogenase occurs in the stomach mucosa; this metabolises ethanol to acetaldehyde and may result in lower levels of ethanol in the portal circulation following ingestion. Lower levels of this enzyme are seen in women and in alcoholics and may increase their susceptibility to developing liver disease.

PATHOPHYSIOLOGY

The mechanism by which alcohol causes liver damage is not clear. Originally it was felt that alcohol itself may not be the causative agent but that associated malnutrition was the required feature along with alcohol excess. This has now been shown not to be the case and attention has focused on the metabolism of ethanol.

During ethanol oxidation, acetaldehyde is formed. It is a highly reactive, labile agent, which may react with hepatocyte components causing damage, or initiate an inflammatory process. Oxygen-derived free radicals may also be generated when ethanol is oxidised by the cytochrome P-450 system and the same reactive species may also promote cellular damage. Endotoxin is produced by intestinal flora and more readily enters the portal circulation owing to increased intestinal permeability; this also enhances the inflammatory response mediated by Kupffer cells within the liver.

CLINICAL FEATURES

History
Having established that the alcohol consumption is excessive and therefore possibly the cause of the liver disease seen in a patient, it is still necessary to consider other aetiologies, and a careful history should be taken for risk factors such as chronic viral hepatitis, haemochromatosis (a relevant family history) and drug use and misuse. Complications of liver disease such as gastrointestinal haemorrhage or the development of ascites should be enquired about, and complications of alcohol abuse that are not related to the liver (Fig. 1) should be discussed.

Examination
This should be specifically focused on features of chronic liver disease but abnormalities may also be detected in virtually any other system. Particular attention should be paid to the patient's mental state, attempting to detect the Wernicke–Korsakoff syndrome or hepatic encephalopathy.

Investigations
Following assessment of the patient, a number of blood tests should be performed as described on pages 78-79. Ultrasound scanning of the abdomen will detect the size and shape of the liver, and any solid tumours that may have developed, the presence of splenomegaly and ascites. Certain common patterns of blood test results are often seen, which point to alcohol abuse with and without liver disease (Table 3).

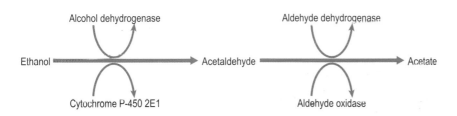

Fig. 2 **Metabolism of alcohol.** At low concentrations, alcohol dehydrogenase metabolises the majority of ethanol; at higher concentrations, the inducible cytochrome P-450 2E1 system, which also metabolises drugs such as paracetamol, operates.

ALCOHOLIC LIVER DISEASE II

LIVER HISTOLOGY

If there is a clear history of alcohol abuse and no evidence of co-existent disease, then biopsy is usually unnecessary. However, when performed, a number of characteristic changes may be seen.

Fatty liver

Fat droplets appear in the cytoplasm of hepatocytes; they may appear a few days after an alcohol binge, but are almost always present in heavy drinkers (> 80 g of alcohol per day for > 5 years). Fatty liver may occur, however, with obesity, diabetes mellitus, starvation and chronic hepatitis C virus infection (Fig. 1).

Alcoholic hepatitis

A combination of the following may occur:

- hepatocyte necrosis with balloon degeneration
- inflammatory infiltrate with neutrophils
- acidophilic bodies representing hepatocyte apoptosis
- Mallory bodies – pink (on H & E stain) intracytoplasmic inclusions
- giant mitochondria in hepatocytes.

Fibrosis/cirrhosis

Fibrosis initially develops adjacent to sinusoids, and then bridges between central veins and portal tracts. Cirrhosis has occurred when there is generalised fibrosis and nodule formation (Fig. 2): when normal relationship between the portal tracts and the central vein is disrupted.

Liver biopsy is usually not necessary in patients with obvious alcohol-related liver disease. It may be necessary when patients deny alcohol consumption and there is doubt, or when other conditions may co-exist, such as iron overload.

MANAGEMENT OF THE ALCOHOLIC WITH DEPRESSED CONSCIOUS LEVEL

This is not an uncommon presentation and there are a number of considerations when evaluating this type of patient.

- First, is the patient simply inebriated and therefore going to recover without any specific therapy? This

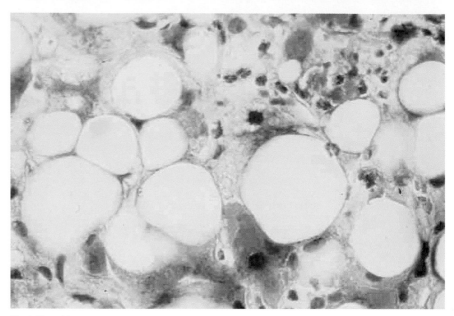
Fig. 1 **Fatty Liver**

may be true but if not and no specific therapy is undertaken when it is required, the patient may die.
- Is there evidence of head injury, raising the possibility of an intracranial haemorrhage? This is more common in alcoholics as they are prone to falling and may be more prone to bleeding if they have abnormal clotting or a low platelet count. Cerebral haemorrhage is also more common in alcohol abuse and CT scan of the brain is necessary to exclude these possibilities.
- Alcoholics often fit and may be in the post-ictal phase when unconscious. A witnessed account, a history of previous fits or evidence of tongue biting or incontinence may be suggestive.
- Hypoglycaemia also occurs frequently and may be a cause of unconsciousness, which can be rapidly excluded by a BM stick.
- Encephalopathy is another possibility and the usual clinical signs should be

sought and treatment instituted.
- Drug overdose should always be considered and a history obtained from witnesses or empty bottles collected from the scene.
- Delirium tremens may occur after a few days of alcohol withdrawal, and may present as depressed conscious level, or with hallucinations and disorientation.

MANAGEMENT OF ALCOHOL WITHDRAWAL

This is another common medical problem and should be recognised and treated promptly. Clinical features of delirium tremens (DTs) start after a few hours of alcohol withdrawal in susceptible individuals with:

- **Insomnia, anxiety, hyperactivity** (5–10 hours after last drink)
- **Tremor, visual or auditory hallucinations, tachycardia and hypertension, fever** (6–30 hours after last drink)

Table 1 **Chlordiazepoxide for alcohol withdrawal**

10 mg × 4 per day (up to a maximum of 100 mg per day) for 2 days
10 mg, 5 mg, 5 mg, 10 mg (8 a.m., 1 p.m., 6 p.m., 11 p.m.) for 2 days
5 mg, 5 mg, 5 mg, 10 mg for 2 days
5 mg, 10 mg (8 a.m., 11 p.m.) for 2 days
10 mg (11 p.m.) for 2 days then stop

This is a guide and doses should be adjusted according to response. Treatment courses should not extend beyond 14 days in view of the risk of addiction.

- **Withdrawal seizures** – 'rum fits' (8–48 hours after last drink)
- **Full-blown DTs – delirium, hallucinations, hypertension, paranoia and clouding of consciousness** (3–5 days after last drink) – may have an associated mortality of up to 15%.

Patients may present with a good history and early features of alcohol withdrawal and should be promptly treated. Occasionally, patients who have been admitted to hospital for another cause, such as an operation, develop full-blown DTs. This should be considered in patients who become acutely confused after being in hospital for a few days.

Treatment should include correction of metabolic abnormalities, administration of thiamine (50 mg i.v. or as an intravenous vitamin combination). Sedation is usually achieved with a benzodiazepine such as chlordiazepoxide, which is given in doses sufficient to control symptoms and is tailed off over 5 days. Dosing should be flexible and adjusted to clinical response, but a typical requirement is outlined in Table 1. An alternative is chlormethiazole infusion, which is effective but requires very careful monitoring to avoid of respiratory depression.

MANAGEMENT OF ALCOHOLIC HEPATITIS

This is a serious complication of alcohol excess and once established may progress despite abstinence. It is characterised by a tachycardia, pyrexia and raised white cell count with deteriorating liver function – a rising bilirubin and lengthening prothrombin time – and is commonly associated with renal dysfunction. It carries a recognised short-term mortality with rapid progression to liver failure or may settle but be a precursor to the development of cirrhosis.

Management depends on complete abstinence from alcohol, careful supportive measures with appropriate fluid and electrolyte balance and prompt treatment of problems such as renal dysfunction, hepatic encephalopathy and gastrointestinal haemorrhage, which may complicate the disease. Oral prednisolone has been shown to improve outcome in patients with severe hepatitis, which is progressing despite abstinence, and in whom infection has been excluded.

MANAGEMENT OF OUTPATIENTS

The ideal management of patients probably includes physician, nurse, counselling service, and social worker. Individuals who are simply abusing alcohol need to be encouraged to moderate their intake, but those who have developed abnormalities of the liver or pancreas should be encouraged to abstain completely, as even modest alcohol intakes can lead to disease progression.

Depression should be recognized and treated; alcohol craving may be helped by naltrexone but aspirin, NSAIDs and paracetamol (which may be toxic in the therapeutic dose range) should be avoided.

Patients with evidence of portal hypertension should be endoscoped and if oesophageal varices are confirmed, they should be prescribed beta-blockers to reduce the risk of haemorrhage.

MANAGEMENT OF ASCITES

This is a common complication in patients with alcoholic liver disease and is dealt with in the context of portal hypertension (p. 88).

HEPATIC ENCEPHALOPATHY

This should be recognised early and the experienced clinician recognises it when present in its most subtle form. When present severely, it should be distinguished from alcohol intoxication (Table 2).

Clinical features include asterixis

Table 2 **Grading of encephalopathy**

1 Mild drowsiness, mild intellectual impairment, rousable and coherent
2 Increased drowsiness with confusion, but rousable
3 Very drowsy and disorientated
4 Comatose, unresponsive or responding to pain only

(slow-frequency flapping tremor), constructional apraxia (failure to copy a five-pointed star), reversed sleep pattern, and hepatic foetor (sweet sickly) breath.

Precipitating factors include biochemical abnormalities such as hyperkalaemia or hyponatraemia, intercurrent infection, ingestion of sedatives, or a high gut protein load as either ingested meat or an upper GI bleed.

The cause should be removed or corrected and treatment is aimed at inducing clearance of the gut. This is usually done with lactulose as it induces defaecation and promotes the production of lactobacilli in the colon, which are less likely to induce encephalopathy.

Magnesium sulphate or lactulose enemas can also be used to promote gut clearance. Neomycin may have a marginal effect in intractable cases.

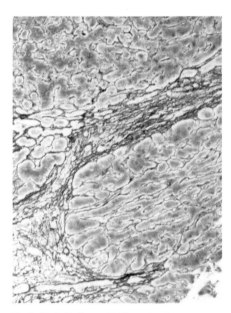

Fig. 2 **Cirrhotic liver with fibrous septae separating nodules of liver tissue.**

Alcoholic liver disease

- Alcohol abuse is a massive international problem which has huge resource implications both for the community as a whole and also for health care.
- Alcohol is enjoyed by many and used safely by the majority of people who drink it.
- Alcohol abuse may be denied or not recognized by individuals or their families and friends.
- Alcohol damages not only the liver, but many other organs also.
- Only 20% of heavy alcohol abusers (> 80 g per day for > 5 years) develop liver disease.

DISORDERS OF IRON AND COPPER METABOLISM

HAEMOCHROMATOSIS

EPIDEMIOLOGY

Haemochromatosis is a genetic condition with autosomal recessive inheritance. In northern European populations up to 1 in 300 individuals are affected. The condition results in excess iron being deposited in the liver, pancreas, joints, pituitary gland and heart, resulting in tissue damage and malfunction.

The gene responsible for haemochromatosis (HFE) has been mapped to chromosome 6, and a single mutation that accounts for the majority of cases (C282Y) has been identified. The frequency of carriage of this gene is approximately 10% in those of northern European descent, and 91% of patients with haemochromatosis are homozygous for this mutation. In southern Europe the proportion of patients homozygous for this mutation is smaller and confirms that the condition is heterogenous.

The mechanism by which this gene causes increased intestinal absorption of iron, which is the primary defect, is not clear.

CLINICAL FEATURES

Age of presentation is usually 40–50 and, although the gene is equally distributed between the sexes, men are more likely to present at this age because women, owing to menstruation, tend to have lower levels of iron overload.

The majority of patients come to light now, either as a result of family screening or as part of an investigation work-up for patients with abnormal liver function tests or liver disease. Early descriptions of the clinical manifestations included pigmentation of the skin and diabetes, the condition originally being termed 'bronzed diabetes'. Now patients present with symptoms that include lethargy, arthralgia, loss of libido or impotence and abdominal pain. Findings include evidence of liver disease or abnormal liver enzymes, skin pigmentation, diabetes (due to iron deposition in the islet cells), feminisation or gynaecomastia in men.

Later presentations include cardiomyopathy with atrial and ventricular dysrhythmias associated with congestive cardiac failure. The arthropathy typically affects the second and third metacarpophalangeal joints, with joint space narrowing and chondrocalcinosis best seen in the knees.

DIAGNOSIS

Iron studies are worth checking in all patients with abnormal liver enzymes, particularly if symp-toms or signs arein keeping with haemochromatosis. The investigations should include measurement of serum ferritin, which is elevated in haemochromatosis. Ferritin levels are raised in other liver diseases, although usually not to the same extent. Iron and transferrin saturation should be calculated (Table 1). CT scanning of the liver can show evidence of iron overload, particularly when this is marked, but lacks sensitivity. MR scanning also detects moderate iron overload but also lacks sensitivity.

Liver biopsy should be undertaken to confirm hepatic iron overload and a quantitative assessment of iron overload can be made. Iron is typically deposited in hepatocytes in the periportal region (Fig. 1). It is also important prognostically, as patients without evidence of liver damage have a normal life expectancy with treatment, whereas in the presence of fibrosis or cirrhosis life expectancy is reduced. Genetic studies are nowroutinely available and patients homozygous for the C282Y mutation are likely to develop iron overload.

MANAGEMENT

Having made the diagnosis, treatment is aimed at reducing total body iron. This is done by regular therapeutic phlebotomy. Each unit (500 ml) of blood contains 250 mg of iron and patients may have as much as 20 g of excess iron, requiring ap-proximately 80 units to be removed This can usually be done weekly to begin with and maintenance is then aimed at keeping this level, with venesection occurring frequently enough to keep a ferritin level below 50 µg/l. This usually requires venesection of 1 unit every 2–3 months.

If patients are diagnosed and treated before significant organ damage has occurred, then life expectancy is normal. Once cirrhosis of the liver has developed, problems related to this and the risk of developing hepatocellular carcinoma

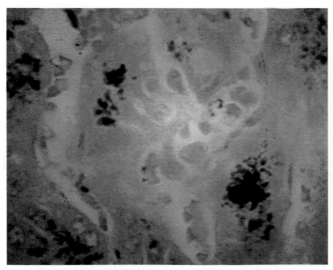

Fig. 1 **Liver biopsy with Perls' stain.**

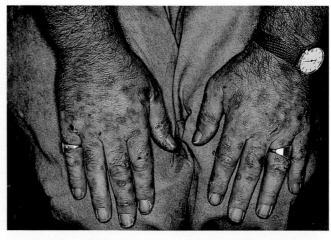

Fig. 2 **Porphyria cutanea tarda.** Changes can be seen on the dorsal aspects of the hands. (Source: Gawkrodger D 2002 Dermatology 3 E, Churchill Livingstone, Edinburgh.

reduce life expectancy. Liver transplantation may be an option in some patients. First-degree relatives should be screened, with measurement of ferritin and iron saturation, and genetic testing. Homozygotes will probably need treatment, as will heterozygotes with abnormal iron studies. Heterozygotes with normal iron studies can just be monitored.

OTHER IRON OVERLOAD STATES

Other liver disorders can cause a rise in ferritin, serum iron, and hepatic iron content. Haemochromatosis is more severe in patients who drink excessive amounts of alcohol, and alcohol abusers without genetic haemochromatosis often have elevated hepatic iron content. A hepatic iron concentration of > 10 000 µ/g is suggestive of haemochromatosis, but younger patients may not have such high liver concentrations, in which case the hepatic iron index may be helpful. The hepatic iron concentration (in µmol/g dry weight) is divided by the age – a value of > 1.9 is consistent with haemochromatosis.

Parenteral iron overload

Patients who require multiple blood transfusion (usually more than 100 units) for haematological disorders or who have chronic increased red cell turnover as in chronic haemolysis (e.g. β thalassaemia) can develop secondary iron overload with iron initially deposited in the Kupffer cells of the liver. Chelation therapy may be necessary to treat this.

Porphyria cutanea tarda

This condition is characterised by photosensitive skin reactions with pigmentation, blistering and scarring (Fig. 2) Unlike acute intermittent porphyria, there are no acute neurological, psychological, or abdominal pain attacks. The condition is associated with alcohol use. Liver enzymes are usually abnormal and hepatic iron overload occurs, causing liver damage which can be complicated by hepatocellular carcinoma. Treatment is effective and is with venesection as for haemochromatosis.

Bantu siderosis

This condition affects South African black people not only in Africa, where porridge and beer prepared in iron pots is thought to be a major contributory factor, but also individuals who have moved from the area, suggesting a genetic predisposition to the iron overload.

WILSON'S DISEASE

Wilson's disease is a rare inherited abnormality of copper metabolism. It is inherited as an autosomal recessive, occurring in 1 : 30 000 live births with an incidence of 30 per million. The gene is distributed worldwide and located on chromosome 13. The 'ATP7B' gene codes for a cation transporting ATPase, and over 40 unique mutations have been described. The abnormality results in reduced incorporation of copper into caeruloplasmin (a copper-binding protein) and subsequent reduced biliary

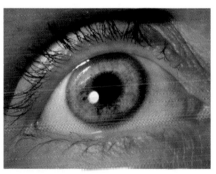
Fig. 3 **Kayser – Fleischer rings.**

excretion of copper. As copper is excreted in bile, cholestatic liver diseases such as primary biliary cirrhosis can lead to increased hepatic deposition of copper.

The average age of presentation is in the teens, and diagnosis after age 40 is rare. Liver abnormalities predominate in childhood with clinical pictures ranging from abnormalities resembling an immune hepatitis to cirrhosis with portal hypertension or acute fulminant hepatic failure. Neurological abnormalities are more common with older presentations and include movement disorders, with rigid dystonias and psychiatric illness.

Diagnosis can be difficult in acute liver failure but depends on demonstrating copper deposition in the cornea (Kayser–Fleischer rings, (Fig. 3) – which may be absent in 25% of patients with just liver abnormalities, a low serum caeruloplasmin, high urinary copper and elevated copper in the liver (Table 2). The condition should be considered in individuals with a hepatitis below the age of 40, particularly when an immune hepatitis or severe drug reaction are the major differentials.

Treatment is with chelating agents such as D-penicillamine and trientine. Zinc may also reduce intestinal absorption. Despite previous concerns regarding teratogenicity, penicillamine should not be discontinued during pregnancy. Screening first-degree relatives should be performed by examining for Kayser–Fleischer rings and measuring serum caeruloplasmin.

Table 2 **Biochemical abnormalities in Wilson's disease**

	Wilson's disease	Normal
Serum caeruloplasmin (mg/l)	0–200	200–350
Serum copper (µmol/l)	3–10	11–24
Urinary copper µmol/day)	> 1.6	< 0.6
Liver copper (µg/g)	> 250	20–50

Catches: Serum caeruloplasmin can be low in fulminant hepatic failure, and various other low protein states, and normal or high in 15% of Wilson's disease patients, particularly during pregnancy and as an acute phase reactant. Care must be taken in obtaining liver samples as contamination can lead to falsely high readings and hepatic copper deposition can be patchy.

Table 1 **Iron studies useful in the diagnosis of haemochromatosis**

	Normal	Haemochromatosis
Ferritin	15–300 ng/ml	Usually > 400 µg/ml
Iron saturation*	16–60%	Usually > 55%

* Equal to the serum iron divided by the total iron-binding capacity

Disorders of iron and copper metabolism

- Haemochromatosis is a common genetic disorder, affecting 1 : 300 in northern Europe, transmitted as an autosomal recessive, associated with iron overload.
- The majority of cases have a gene defect (C282Y) on chromosome 6.
- Diagnosis depends on demonstrating iron overload, and the condition is best screened for with a serum ferritin assay.
- Other conditions can cause a raised level of ferritin in the serum and excessive iron deposition in the liver.
- Wilson's disease is a rare genetic disorder, transmitted as an autosomal recessive, associated with copper overload.
- The defect has been mapped to chromosome 13.
- Treatment requires chelation therapy.

INHERITED AND INFILTRATIVE DISORDERS

DISORDERS OF BILIRUBIN METABOLISM

Gilbert's syndrome

This is a common inherited abnormality of bilirubin metabolism giving rise to a modest elevation in the serum bilirubin (Fig. 1). It is probably inherited as an autosomal dominant and affects approximately 5% of the population. It often presents in adolescence when a family member notices a mild degree of jaundice, or the hyperbilirubinaemia is picked up on routine testing for another reason, such as pretreatment testing for acne.

The serum bilirubin is not usually elevated above 80 μmol/l and a moderate proportion of this is unconjugated. The gamma glutamyl transpeptidase (GGT) and transaminases are normal, as is the hepatic alkaline phosphatase, but because these patients are often diagnosed in their youth, the bony alkaline phosphatase may be elevated, due to active growth.

Individuals are usually asymptomatic but may experience some mild right upper quadrant discomfort. The jaundice is most noticeable during intercurrent illnesses such as colds or flu and may be worsened during periods of starvation.

There is a defect in the glucuronidation of bilirubin in the liver which leads to a rise in unconjugated bilirubin. Unfortunately, a request for this proportion to be assayed by the laboratory, often elicits a result that is quoted as a 'direct' or 'indirect' value. This is due to the way

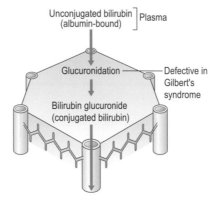

Fig. 1 **Metabolic defect causing elevated serum levels of bilirubin.**

in which bilirubin is assayed and requires the clinician to remember that direct bilirubin is conjugated and that indirect represents the unconjugated fraction. On examination, the individual is normal apart from perhaps a tinge of jaundice but, in particular, there should be no stigmata of chronic liver disease.

Investigation requires exclusion of haemolysis with a normal blood film and serum haptoglobin concentration, and confirmation that other routine liver tests are normal. No further investigation is required and an explanation is all that is necessary to the individual or the parents. It should be pointed out that the condition has no bearing on life expectancy, will not predispose to other conditions and can be considered a variation of normal.

Crigler–Najjar syndrome

Type 1

A much rarer cause of elevated unconju-gated bilirubin, this presents as neonatal jaundice, is inherited as an autosomal recessive, and is due to an absence of conjugating enzyme. Death due to kernicterus is usually in early childhood.

Type 2

This is also inherited as an autosomal recessive but with incomplete absence of conjugating enzyme so that survival to adulthood occurs. There is severe unconjugated hyperbilirunaemia and treatment with phototherapy or phenobarbitone to induce hepatic enzymes helps.

Dubin–Johnson syndrome

This rare, autosomal recessive condition results in elevated bilirubin which is predominately conjugated, and is due to defective excretion of conjugated bile. All other routine liver tests are normal. There is a characteristic black discoloration of the liver and no serious sequelae of the condition. Jaundice may be worsened by oral oestrogens and these should be avoided.

Rotor syndrome

Like Dubin–Johnson syndrome, this results in a mild rise in conjugated bilirubin, has no effect on survival and requires no treatment. There is no black discoloration of the liver.

OTHER INHERITED DISORDERS

α₁-Antitrypsin deficiency

α_1-Antitrypsin (α_1-AT) is the major hepatic protease inhibitor, and is produced almost exclusively in the liver. It

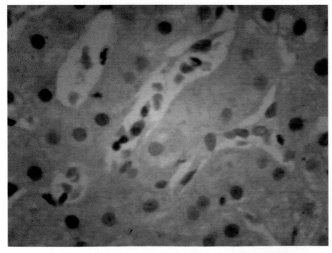

Fig. 2 **Liver biopsy with apple green birefringence in amyloid disease.**

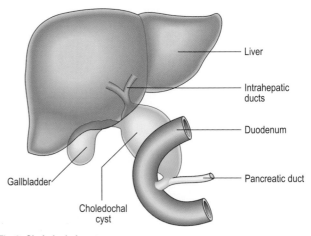

Fig. 3 **Choledochal cyst.**

binds with, and deactivates elastase. A defect of excretion of α_1-AT occurs and is inherited as an autosomal recessive, but with codominant expression. Homozygous deficiency occurs in 1:1500 in Europe and with similar frequency in the USA. Homozygotes for the condition are prone to developing cirrhosis and emphysema of the lung, particularly if they drink or smoke respectively. Primary hepatocellular cancer is also more common. Heterozygotes may also develop liver disease.

Neonates may present with liver disease, or adults with cirrhosis at an early stage. Because α_1-AT is an acute phase reactant, phenotyping studies should be undertaken. Normal allelic representation is protease inhibitor MM (PiMM), and the homozygote is PiZZ.

Liver biopsy shows characteristic PAS-positive, diastase-negative globules associated with a hepatitis or cirrhosis.

Treatment is supportive, with portal hypertension and ascites treated conventionally. Liver transplantation may be necessary to cure the underlying defect.

INBORN ERRORS OF METABOLISM

GLYCOGEN STORAGE

There is a group of inherited disorders of glycogen metabolism, each one related to a defect in a different step of the pathway. The conditions usually present in childhood and are characterised by hypoglycaemia, as hepatic glycogen cannot be adequately mobilised to glucose when absorbed glucose from the gut is insufficient to maintain blood sugar. Owing to the vast amounts of hepatic glycogen, there is marked hepatomegaly. Diagnosis depends on demonstrating excess hepatic glycogen with specific enzyme defects measured in vitro.

LIPID STORAGE

Gaucher's disease

This is a rare autosomal recessive disease to which Ashkenazi Jews are prone. Owing to a defect in glucocerebrosidase, glucocerebroside accumulates in reticuloendothelial cells, particularly in the liver, bone marrow and spleen. This results in bone fractures due to bone cysts and hepatosplenomegaly. There is skin pigmentation and pingueculae (yellow thickenings on either side of the pupil). Diagnosis depends on demonstrating characteristic foamy cells with pale cytoplasm' 'Gaucher cells,' in the bone marrow, and β-glucocerebrosidase can be measured in mononuclear cells in the blood. Treatment is with infusions of replacement enzyme.

Niemann–Pick disease

This is another rare autosomal recessive disease which is more common in Jewish populations. There is a defect in the metabolism of sphingomyelin resulting in its accumulation in the lysosomes of reticuloendothelial cells. This causes massive hepatosplenomegaly in childhood. There is a characteristic cherry red spot on the macula. Diagnosis depends on demonstrating typical Niemann–Pick cells in the marrow, and treatment has been with bone marrow transplantation.

LIVER INFILTRATION

AMYLOID

This condition is frequently a differential diagnosis of hepatomegaly. The characteristic of the condition is deposition of glycoprotein — either AA type, which can occur as a result of chronic inflammatory conditions such as rheumatoid arthritis or inflammatory bowel disease, or the rarer AL type, which can occur in the absence of other diseases although is associated with myeloma.

Amyloid protein is deposited in the spleen, kidneys and liver, resulting in organ enlargement. There tends to be little hepatic dysfunction although portal hypertension may occasionally occur.

Diagnosis can be made by subcutaneous fat pad aspiration, rectal biopsy demonstrating apple green birefringence or liver biopsy (Fig. 2). This can be hazardous as haemorrhage is more common from the amyloid-infiltrated liver.

The outlook is poor with a majority dieing within 2 years of diagnosis. Treatment is aimed at the underlying condition in AA amyloid, and melphalan and prednisolone may help in AL amyloid.

Hepatobiliary cystic disease

A rare group of congenital cystic diseases of the liver and biliary tree exist. Cystic dilatation of the biliary tree can occur leading to a dilated common bile duct (choledochal cyst) (Fig. 3). Variations can occur with dilatation occurring up into the hepatic ducts, or right down into the intramucosal portion of the distal CBD (choledochocele). If there are intrahepatic duct cysts alone it is termed Caroli's disease (Fig. 4). The liver histology is normal but patients develop intrahepatic stones and sepsis. The intrahepatic duct cysts can be associated with congenital hepatic fibrosis and the term Caroli's syndrome then applies.

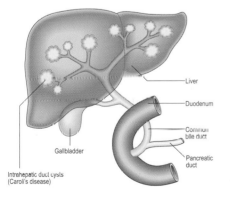

Intrahepatic duct cysts
(Caroli's disease)
Liver
Duodenum
Common bile duct
Gallbladder
Pancreatic duct

Fig. 4 **Caroli's disease.**

Inherited and infiltrative disorders

- Gilbert's syndrome affects around 5% of the population and is characterised by mild unconjugated hyperbilirubinaemia, with normal LFTs.
- It is does not predispose to other liver diseases and does not affect life expectancy.
- Glycogen storage diseases are rare and usually present in childhood with hypoglycaemia and hepatomegaly.
- Lipid storage diseases are more common amongst Jewish races and present in childhood with hepatosplenomegaly.
- Amyloid disease is a rare condition that results from deposition of amyloid in various organs and can complicate chronic inflammatory conditions or arise as a primary disease.

PORTAL HYPERTENSION I

ANATOMY AND PATHOPHYSIOLOGY

The portal vein is formed by the confluence of the splenic vein, the superior mesenteric vein (SMV) and the inferior mesenteric vein (IMV). The splenic vein drains the spleen and the tail of the pancreas. The SMV drains the small intestine, the colon to the splenic flexure and the head of the pancreas. The IMV drains the rest of the colon and rectum (Fig. 1). Normal portal blood flow is 1–1.2 l/min and the portal pressure is 7 mmHg. Hepatic artery flow is just 0.4 l/min with a pressure of 100 mmHg. The hepatic vein flow is 1.6 l/min with the same pressure as in the inferior vena cava of 4 mmHg. Although the oxygen content of the portal blood is relatively low compared to that of the hepatic artery (and gets lower during digestion), the high blood flow means that it actually provides ~ 70% of the hepatic oxygen supply.

Portal pressure in cirrhosis rises to about 18 mmHg and needs to be above 12 mmHg for oesophageal varices to develop. As a result of these pressure rises, blood shunts at points of portal–systemic anastomoses. This increased blood flow causes veins to distend, producing varices (Table 1). There is also congestion of the spleen, resulting in splenomegaly, and of the GI tract, resulting in congestion of the mucosa of the gut (Fig. 2).

Hepatic venography allows measurement of the free hepatic vein pressure and also a 'wedged' hepatic vein pressure. A catheter with a balloon and distal pressure monitor is wedged into a hepatic vein radical and the balloon inflated. The difference between wedged and free pressures reflects the sinusoidal venous pressure. In presinusoidal causes of portal hypertension there is usually a low wedged pressure.

Portal pressure can be measured via a transhepatic catheter into the portal vein.

CAUSES OF PORTAL HYPERTENSION

There are many causes of portal hypertension and because chronic liver disease is the commonest it is easy to forget the other causes. Portal hypertension usually occurs as a result of impairment of flow of blood along the course of the portal vein. This may occur in the portal vein itself 'prehepatic', within the liver 'intrahepatic', or finally in the hepatic vein or its tributaries 'post-hepatic'.

Prehepatic causes

Portal vein thrombosis

This presents with features of portal hypertension but sometimes without features of chronic liver disease. There is splenomegaly and features of hypersplenism, but without hepatomegaly or liver dysfunction. Haemorrhage from oesophageal varices occurs and may be the presenting feature. Liver decompensation with encephelopathy tends not to occur if there is no significant pre-existing liver disease. Ascites may occur transiently at the time of the thrombosis, but tends to settle spontaneously as collaterals develop.

The condition may occur spontaneously, particularly in patients with coagulopathy (such as protein C deficiency), may follow trauma, or complicate malignancies such as

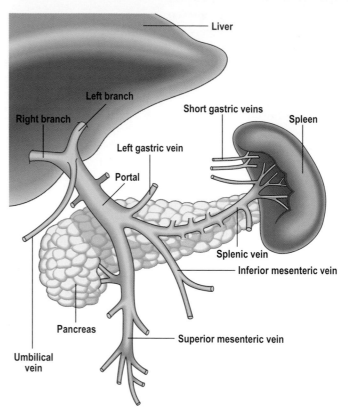

Fig. 1 **The anatomy of the portal venous system.**

Table 1 **Portal – systemic collaterals in portal hypertension**

Anastamotic site (portal – systemic anastomosis)	Result
Left gastric and short gastric/intercostal and oesophageal veins	Gastro-oesophageal varices
Superior haemorrhoidal/inferior haemorrhoidal	Rectal varices
Umbilical vein/anterior abdominal wall veins	Caput medusae*
Splenorenal ligament to left kidney	Splenorenal varices
Abdominal organ veins/retroperitoneal venous system	Retroperitoneal varices

* Do not develop when the cause of portal hypertension is proximal to the umbilical vein joining the portal vein.

Table 2 **Causes of portal vein thrombosis**

Hypercoagulable states
Antiphospholipid syndrome
Factor V mutations
Myeloproliferative disease
Protein C/S deficiency

Inflammatory diseases
Crohn's disease
Pancreatitis
Ulcerative colitis

Iatrogenic
Following liver transplantation
Following splenectomy
Following umbilical catheterisation

Infections
Appendicitis
Diverticulitis
Liver diseases
Cirrhosis
Nodular regenerative hyperplasia
Hepatocellular carcinoma

hepatocellular carcinoma or local invasion of the portal vein by pancreatic cancer (Table 2). Children may develop portal vein thrombosis following infection of the umbilical vein, which occurs in the neona-

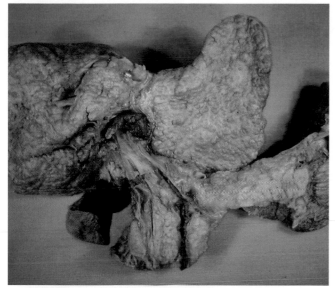

Fig. 2 **Post mortem specimen of cirrhotic liver and enlarged spleen.**

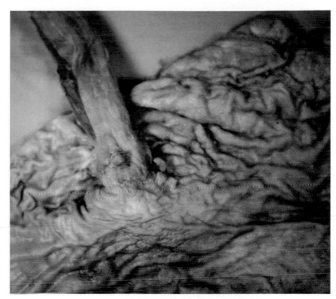

Fig. 4 **Post mortem specimen of banded oesophageal varix.**

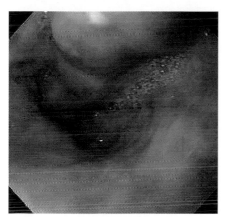

Fig. 3 **Oesophageal varices at endosurgery.**

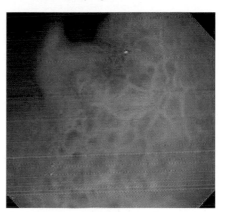

Fig. 5 **Portal hypertensive gastropathy at endosurgery.**

Increased blood flow because of massive splenomegaly

Occasionally there is such massive blood flow through an enlarged, diseased spleen that this results in portal hypertension. In these circumstances, splenectomy may be helpful. Beta blockade will not help.

Intrahepatic causes

The perisinusoidal causes are rarer and include primary biliary cirrhosis in which, at least in part, there is perisinusoidal portal hypertension, and schistosomiasis where there is a reaction in the terminal portal venules.

Cirrhosis

Cirrhosis, regardless of aetiology, causes portal hypertension. This occurs as blood in the portal vein is directed around nodules, impeding blood flow, and as portal veins form anastomoses with hepatic veins, bypassing hepatic sinusoids.

OESOPHAGEAL AND GASTRIC VARICES

The development of oesophageal or gastric varices as a result of portal hypertension is a serious development and should be sought when portal hypertension is suspected. Detection is best done at endoscopy performed by an experienced endoscopist. Oesophageal varices are seen as distended tortuous veins in the distal oesophagus and are usually readily recognised (Figs 3 and 4), whilst gastric varices occur in the gastric fundus and may be mistaken for normal gastric folds. A common reason for oesophageal varices to be missed is that bleeding has occurred with a drop in the portal pressure, causing the varices to collapse. Portal hypertensive gastropathy is usually present (Fig. 5),

tal period and is particularly common in India.

If the acute episode presents with haemorrhage from oeophageal varices, then conventional treatment with banding or sclerotherapy is necessary. Anticoagulation is usually too late, even in the acute presentation of portal vein thrombosis, and is contraindicated in patients who are bleeding. Surgical shunting is not usually possible. More commonly, the condition is diagnosed following the discovery of portal hypertension, in which case beta blockade should be instituted. Diagnosis can be made with colour flow Doppler at ultrasound scanning (which demonstrates no portal venous flow) venography or MR imaging.

Once the patient is stable, the underlying condition should be sought and treated.

Splenic vein thrombosis

This usually follows pancreatic diseases such as pancreatitis or carcinoma and may result in varices in the fundus of the stomach but few in the oesophagus. Splenectomy, by removing arterial supply, is curative.

which should encourage the endoscopist to search particularly thoroughly for varices.

Once varices have been detected, patients should be given a non-selective beta-blocker such as propranolol. The clinician should aim for a reduction of 25% in the resting pulse rate, which leads to a fall in the portal pressure and consequent reduction in the risk of bleeding. Unfortunately, up to 25% of patients are intolerant of beta blockade. Initiation of treatment with propranolol should not be until the acute haemorrhage has been securely controlled.

If varices are detected at endoscopy for diagnosis of upper GI haemorrhage, then endoscopic therapy should be undertaken. If bleeding is difficult to control, patients should be started on an infusion that may help to reduce portal pressure, such as somatostatin or terlipressin. There is speculation that the presence of endotoxin released from gut bacteria causes portal pressure to rise enough to induce haemorrhage from oesophageal varices. Consequently, it may be helpful to start all patients who are actively bleeding on an antibiotic such as ciprofloxacin.

PORTAL HYPERTENSION II

Sclerotherapy for oesophageal varices

This technique is being superseded by banding but is still widely used and has a place in controlling active bleeding where only poor views are obtainable. A sclerotherapy needle is placed via the channel of the endoscope directly into the varix, which is injected with 1–2 ml of a sclerosant such as ethanolamine oleate. Paravariceal injection into the submucosa may also be effective in stemming haemorrhage but has a higher risk of sclerotherapy complications such as mucosal ulceration and chemical mediastinitis. The procedure is usually repeated every 7–10 days until the varices are ablated. Subsequent mucosal ulceration and strictures may develop.

Banding for oesophageal varices

This is a similar technique to that used with haemorrhoids. An applicator is placed on the end of the endoscope (Fig. 1), varices are sucked into this applicator and the mechanism fired, which releases a small rubber band around the varix (Fig. 2). The varix thromboses and over the next 7–10 days the band falls off leaving a small scar where the varix had been. The technique is rapid and a number of bands can be applied in one go. It appears to be less frequently associated with adverse effects than sclerotherapy and is effective at rapidly ablating varices, usually within two to three sessions. An interval of 2 or 3 weeks between treatments is usual, to allow time for the bands to drop off.

Varices in the gastric fundus are more difficult to treat in that conventional sclerosing agents are ineffective and acrylic glue has to be used, which fills the varix and prevents bleeding.

If it proves impossible to control haemorrhage with a combination of a vasoactive drug and endoscopic therapy, then a Sengstaken–Blakemore tube can be inserted, which allows tamponade at the gastro-oesophageal junction, reducing variceal blood flow (Fig. 2). If this fails, oesophageal transection may be undertaken or portal pressure may be reduced by placement

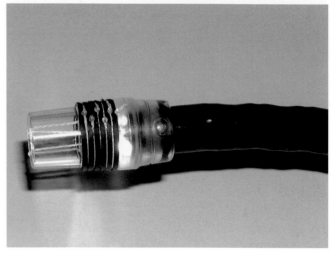

Fig. 1 **Banding introducer on gastroscope**

of a transjugular intrahepatic portosystemic shunt (TIPS), whereby the radiologist places a stent via the jugular vein into the liver, creating a shunt between the low-pressure hepatic venous system and the high-pressure portal venous system. Unfortunately, although this is effective in controlling acute haemorrhage, it can lead to intractable encephelopathy as blood is shunted past the liver. In the longer term a high proportion of shunts close, such that severe portal hypertension returns.

ASCITES

Ascites develops as a result of a combination of circumstances including:

- sodium and water retention by the kidney owing to hyperaldosteronism
- reduction in the plasma osmotic pressure because of low plasma albumin
- increased hepatic lymph flow through the thoracic duct
- dilatation of the splanchnic vascular bed
- portal hypertension.

There is total body water and sodium excess. Once ascites has developed, there is a 50% mortality within 2 years, and once ascites has become resistant to treatment, 50% die within 6 months.

If ascites has developed as a result of portal hypertension, it is usually possible to demonstrate other evidence of portal hypertension such as varices and splenomegaly. There is usually evidence of liver disease, but there may not be, depending on the aetiology of the portal hypertension.

A diagnostic paracentesis is safe and essential, in order to exclude spontaneous bacterial peritonitis, which may occur in up to 30% of patients with ascites. Samples should be sent for culture, but a WBC count greater than 500/mm^3 or neutrophil count of over 250/mm^3 is suggestive of infection. This requires treatment with either a third-generation cephalosporin or an aminoquinolone, such as ciprofloxacin.

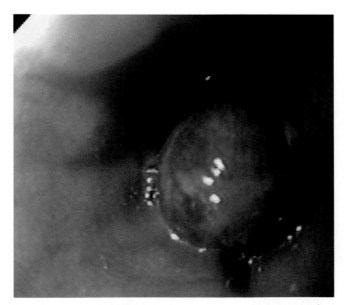

Fig. 2 **Banded oesophageal varix.**

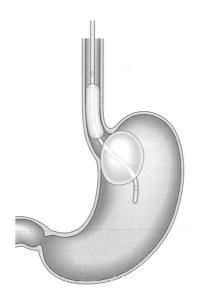

Fig. 3 **Positioning of a Sengstaken–Blakemore tube in situ.**

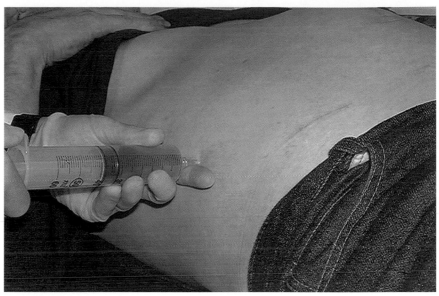

Fig. 4 **Diagnostic paracentesis.**

A serum–ascitic fluid albumin gradient of > 11 g/l is highly suggestive of portal hypertension. An exudate may occur if there is superadded infection, malignancy, or hepatic vein thrombosis.

Patients should be placed on a salt-restricted diet, 40–60 mmol per day if possible but this is rather unpalatable and 88 mmol per day may be more acceptible.

Spironolactone 100 mg per day is usually started as this antagonises the hyperaldosteronism that occurs in chronic liver disease. This is adjusted according to response, up to 400 mg per day. Generally, loop diuretics should be avoided, but a low dose of bumetanide is often effective in initiating a diuresis. There is often a degree of inertia in initating the mobilisation of ascitic fluid, but once the patient's weight starts to fall it is often necessary to reduce the diuretics. The diuretics may induce hyponatraemia without attaining a suitable diuresis, in which case fluid restriction down to 1 l per day may be necessary.

Biochemistry should be closely monitored as over-diuresis can lead to encephalopathy and renal failure, and weight reduction of 0.5 kg per day should be aimed for (Fig. 5).

Ascites is refractory when diuretics and salt restriction fail to clear the ascites, or the complications of treatment (encephalopathy, rising creatinine, hyponatraemia, or hypo- or hyperkalaemia) prevent adequate fluid clearance.

Therapeutic (complete) paracentesis can be performed in patients with stable liver and renal function. A large-bore drainage catheter is placed, using strict aseptic technique. Simultaneous intravenous infusion of salt-poor albumin (8 g per litre of fluid removed) or colloid is undertaken to prevent vascular collapse.

Resistant ascites can be treated with a TIPS procedure, but despite an early response, ascites frequently recurs and encephalopathy commonly complicates the procedure. Liver transplantation may also be considered in these patients. In patients in whom the ascites cannot be completely cleared, it is useful to maintain them on an aminoquinolone such as norfloxacin in order to prevent the development of bacterial peritonitis.

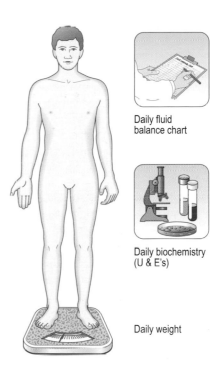

Daily fluid balance chart

Daily biochemistry (U & E's)

Daily weight

Fig. 5 **Monitoring of patients with ascites.**

Portal hypertension

- Normal portal vein pressure is 7 mmHg and pressure is usually above 12 mmHg when oesophageal varices develop.
- The majority of the oxygen supply of the liver comes from the portal vein, owing to its high flow compared to that in the hepatic artery.
- Portal hypertension has prehepatic, intrahepatic and post-hepatic causes.
- Patients with stable portal hypertension should be given beta-blockers.
- Treatment of ascites requires both dietary salt restriction and diuretics.
- Fluid restriction is only necessary if hyponatraemia develops.
- Spontaneous bacterial peritonitis is common in patients with ascites and requires detection and treatment.

CHOLESTATIC LIVER DISEASES

PRIMARY BILIARY CIRRHOSIS

Primary biliary cirrhosis (PBC) was first described as a condition that predominantely affected middle-aged women, with jaundice, pruritus and xanthomas. This was largely the clinical presentation of the condition up until the last 30 or 40 years. It remains a condition which mostly affects women – only 15% or so of patients with PBC are men – but the condition is now often diagnosed in the asymptomatic phase.

EPIDEMIOLOGY

There are geographic variations worldwide with a prevalence in the UK of approximately 100 per million of population. Worldwide variations are not adequately explained, but environmental factors may play a part. One study from Sheffield, UK demonstrated that the prevalence of PBC in one area was 10 times that of surrounding areas served by different water reservoirs within the same city. No bacterial or chemical explanation for this has been found despite vigorous investigation.

In 95% of cases of PBC, antimitochondrial antibodies are demonstrated (in titres > 1:40) which are directed against part of the pyruvate dehydrogenase complex on the inner membrane of mitochondria. This shares antigenic similarities with Gram-negative bacteria, and it has been suggested that organisms from either the gut or the urinary tract in some way trigger the immune response that causes the liver damage. However, PBC damage is mediated by T cells, and antimitochondrial anti-

bodies are probably not injurious. There appears to be a familial predisposition, as there is a prevalence of 4–6% amongst first-degree relatives. It remains unclear why the majority affected are women.

PATHOLOGY

In PBC there is an intense inflammatory response focused on bile ducts, resulting eventually in bile duct destruction. The portal inflammatory cells are predominately CD3 positive T lymphocytes. As the bile ducts are destroyed, granulomas commonly form at the site of the damaged duct and represent a characteristic feature of PBC. In response to bile duct loss there is bile ductule regeneration. Fibrosis develops between portal zones and subsequently cirrhosis may develop (Table 1). There may be a non-specific rise in liver copper, which occurs in cholestatic diseases.

SEROLOGY

Only a small proportion of patients with PBC have negative antimitochondrial antibodies (AMA), but AMA is not specific for PBC. The specificity has been increased with subtyping – M2 antibodies, which react with antigens on the inner mitochondrial membrane, are present in 98%.

CLINICAL FEATURES

The condition presents predominantly in women aged 30–60 and may be picked up following routine liver tests, or the patient may present with pruritus, jaundice or complications of portal hypertension. The blood picture shows a cholestatic pattern with initially just elevation in the levels of AP and GGT.

Later, as the disease progresses, the bilirubin level rises, but changes in the aminotransferases are usually modest.

AMA testing is usually positive and the IgM is elevated in 90% of patients. Hypercholesterolaemia is a common feature but there does not appear to be an increased risk of atherosclerotic disease in patients with PBC. Examination may be normal or show a pigmented woman with hepatomegaly and xanthelasma (Fig. 1). Ultrasound examination demonstrates no obstruction. Liver biopsy can be performed, which will help stage the condition, but in a well patient with mild liver changes and positive AMA, the risk associated with biopsy may be unjustifiable.

Progression of the condition is unpredictable, although in asymptomatic patients who are discovered to have PBC in later life, it tends to run an indolent course. Patients may, however, progress inexorably towards end-stage cirrhosis and liver transplantation. The condition in men, although rare, behaves in a similar fashion. Having established that cholestatic LFTs are not due to obstruction, the differential diagnosis is relatively straightforward (Table 2).

ASSOCIATIONS

A number of extrahepatic disorders of immune origin are associated with PBC. These include rheumatological disorders such as Sjögren's syndrome and Raynaud's phenomenon, thyroid disease, and coeliac disease. Osteomalacia may be present at diagnosis owing to vitamin D malabsorption, but osteoporosis is much more common.

MANAGEMENT

Ursodeoxycholic acid (UDCA) is a nonnative bile acid which is more hydrophilic than human bile acids and replaces them in the bile pool. Treatment with UDCA improves biochemical parameters in PBC, but evidence that it has an effect on the liver histology has been more difficult to demonstrate. There is, however, a suggestion that UDCA treatment delays the requirement for liver transplantation by up to 2 years. The UDCA dose is 10–15 mg/kg and treatment seems to be most effective when started early. LFTs appear to improve and often normalise over the

Table 1 **Descriptive stages of PBC histology**

Stage	Feature
1	Florid bile duct lesions
2	Ductular proliferation
3	Scarring (septal fibrosis and bridging)
4	Cirrhosis

Table 2 **Differential diagnosis for PBC**

	Clinical features	AMA	Liver biopsy
PBC	Female, pruritus, raised AP	+	Bile duct damage, ductular proliferation, granulomas
Primary sclerosing cholangitis	Males, UC associated	– or low titre	Ductular proliferation, onion skin duct fibrosis
Sarcoid	Equal sexes	–	Granulomas
Cholestatic drug reactions	Equal sexes History of drug exposure		Portal reaction with granulomas

first few months of treatment and itch will usually improve. Itch, however, can be a major difficulty and treatment with cholestyramine, rifampicin or corticosteroids may all be helpful. Problems with bone disease and corticosteroids make these largely unacceptable. Antihistamines are usually ineffective in helping itch.

Bone disease should be specifically sought and treated. Hormone replacement therapy (HRT) may be acceptable to prevent further bone loss in post menopausal women, but close monitoring of LFTs should be undertaken and HRT discontinued if there are signs of deterioration. Bisphosphonates should be considered.

Portal hypertension once recognised should be treated with propranolol, and spironolactone can be used for the treatment of ascites.

Liver transplantation has now become a widely accepted treatment for advanced PBC. 1-year survival figures for PBC after transplantation are now over 90%, and 8-year survival has been reported at 70%. A rising level of bilirubin is associated with decreased patient survival and once the serum concentration has reached 100 μmol/l, patients should be referred to a liver transplant centre. Patients with Child–Pugh class B or C disease and those having particular problems with portal hypertension or ascites should also be referred. It is not entirely clear what proportion of transplanted livers develop PBC but this does appear to occur in some.

PRIMARY SCLEROSING CHOLANGITIS

Primary sclerosing cholangitis (PSC) is rarer than PBC, but is a progressive cholestatic liver disease of probable immune origin. 70% of sufferers are male and at least 70% of patients with PSC have inflammatory bowel disease, usually ulcerative colitis (UC). The condition may present prior to the development of UC which usually follows a benign course. There is increased frequency of HLA-B8, -DR2 and -DR3.

PATHOLOGY

There is portal tract enlargement with oedema and increased connective tissue resulting in fibrous obliterative cholangitis of bile ducts of all sizes – early stages may appear 'onion-skin'–like on histology. Bile

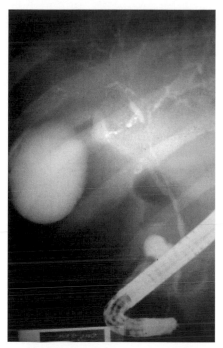

Fig. 1 **Spidery bile ducts of primary sclerosing cholangitis shown at ERCP.**

duct proliferation also occurs.

CLINICAL FEATURES

Patients usually present in their 40s with pruritus or bacterial cholangitis. Most commonly, however, the condition is picked up on routine liver screening in patients with inflammatory bowel disease. The blood picture shows chronic cholestasis with elevated alkaline phosphatase and GGT and in more advanced cases a raised level of bilirubin. Unlike PBC, autoantibodies are not diagnostically helpful.

DIAGNOSIS

Although the histology of PSC is relatively characteristic, changes may be patchy and diagnosis is based on typical appearances at cholangiography (Fig. 1). There is dif-

fuse stricturing and beading of intra- and extrahepatic bile ducts, which may be widespread or, on occasion, occur as a single large duct stricture.

ASSOCIATIONS

Apart from the association between UC and PSC, there is an increased risk of cholangiocarcinoma in patients with PSC and a particularly increased risk of colon cancer in this group. Patients with PSC have problems with fat-soluble vitamin absorption similar to those of patients with PBC and are also prone to bone disease.

MANAGEMENT

Because of the irregular narrowing that occurs in the biliary tree in PSC, areas of bile stasis occur and are prone to become infected causing cholangitis. A deterioration in LFTs with a pyrexia and rigors requires prompt treatment with antibiotics. Oral ciprofloxacin gives high biliary concentrations and good cover against Gram-negative organisms. Prophylactic therapy with ciprofloxacin may be appropriate in patients who regularly experience episodes of bacterial cholangitis.

Endoscopic therapy (dilatation and stenting) for dominant lesions in the large bile ducts also has a place.

UDCA is also used in the treatment of PSC but again the evidence for its long-term benefit is scant.

Liver transplantation is performed for advanced PSC, although biliary strictures may recur, and patients seem prone to developing chronic ductopenic rejection.

Because of the increased risk of colon cancer in patients with PSC and UC, colonic surveillance should be started earlier than in patients with UC alone

Cholestatic liver diseases

- PBC is a condition that predominately affects women and may present with itch, jaundice and xanthelasma, but now is more commonly detected by multichannel screening, demonstrating cholestatic LFTs.
- Patients have elevated alkaline phosphatase and GGT, a positive antimitochondrial antibody test (particularly M2 type) and raised IgM.
- UDCA improves blood results and may delay progression. Liver transplantation should be considered when portal hypertension or its consequences are difficult to control, or the bilirubin has risen above 100 μmol/l.
- PSC is associated with ulcerative colitis, and presents with persistently abnormal LFTs, jaundice or cholangitis.
- Diagnosis is best made at ERCP.
- UDCA may be helpful, as may endoscopic treatment of dominant lesions.

OBSTRUCTIVE JAUNDICE

Obstructive jaundice is a common form of presentation in the older age group and the characteristic features of pale stool, dark urine and itch should always point to this. A markedly raised level of alkaline phosphatase, bilirubin and gamma glutamyl transpeptidase (GGT), with dilated common bile or intrahepatic ducts, confirms obstruction. The commonest causes of this clinical picture are common bile duct (CBD) stones (which have been dealt with on p. 00), carcinoma of the head of the pancreas and bile duct cancers or cholangiocarcinomas. Occasionally, chronic pancreatitis can cause distal CBD strictures which can be difficult to differentiate from early pancreatic cancers.

CARCINOMA OF THE PANCREAS

Carcinoma of the pancreas is more common in men (2 : 1), is the fourth most common cause of cancer death in men, and usually presents when patients are in their 60s or 70s. There is an increased risk of developing the condition in patients who have familial pancreatitis, cigarette smokers, patients with gallstones and those who abuse alcohol. 60% of tumours arise in the head of the pancreas, which commonly causes jaundice, whilst tumours in the body and tail do this less frequently and usually present with pain.

CLINICAL FEATURES

The common presentation is with jaundice, pruritus, a mild nagging epigastric pain which often radiates through to the back and weight loss. These symptoms may occur together or individually, and present a diagnostic conundrum, particularly if patients merely present with weight loss. Occasionally, patients present with a thrombosis due to the hypercoagulable state that often accompanies this malignancy; they may have a deep vein thrombosis in the leg or a more unusual thrombosis such as of the axillary vein. Examination can reveal a jaundiced, cachectic patient with excoriations. There may be a palpable gallbladder (Courvoisier's sign) or abdominal mass. Occasionally, infiltration of the tumour into the duodenum causes vomiting due to gastric outlet obstruction.

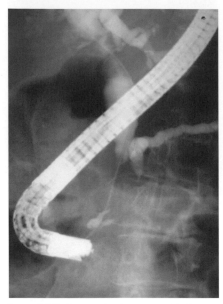

Fig. 1 **ERCP showing distal stricture of CBD and pancreatic duct.**

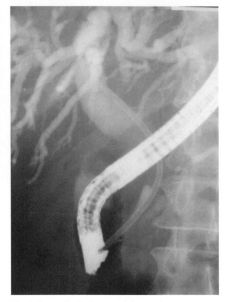

Fig. 2 **Stented carcinoma of the pancreas.**

INVESTIGATIONS

Liver function tests (LFTs) reveal an obstructive picture with raised levels of alkaline phosphatase, bilirubin and GGT. Ultrasound of the biliary tree reveals a dilated CBD and intrahepatic ducts if the tumour is in the head of the pancreas, and may reveal a mass in advanced cases.

Obstructive jaundice is less likely to occur in tumours of the body and tail of the pancreas. ERCP may reveal duodenal invasion by tumour but is most useful in demonstrating an obstructed CBD with a distal stricture (Fig. 1). It is also possible to place a stent at the time of ERCP (Fig. 2), which allows bile drainage, and obtain brushings or biopsies to aid diagnosis. CT scanning may demonstrate smaller tumours than are demonstrable by ultrasound, but is best performed prior to stenting as the prosthesis creates artefacts; it also allows demonstration of local invasion or distant metastases (Fig. 3).

Diagnostic difficulties occur when the tumour is small and not visualised on CT, and raise the question of whether the obstruction is due to a small pancreatic tumour or a benign stricture such as may occur following chronic pancreatitis. Serological testing may be helpful with assay of CA19-9, a carbohydrate marker which rises with some but not all pancreatic tumours. A mass, if present, can be biopsied under ultrasound or CT guidance for confirmation.

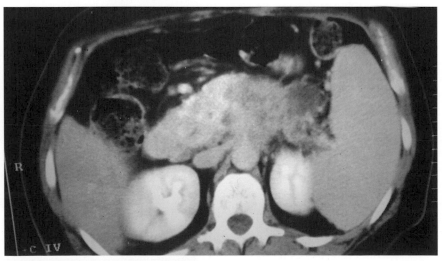

Fig. 3 **CT scan of carcinoma of the pancreas.**

MANAGEMENT

The only hope of cure for pancreatic cancer is surgical resection. For patients to be operable they should be generally fit and there should be no evidence of local invasion, particularly into surrounding vessels, nor should there be distant metastases. A Whipple's procedure carries an operative mortality of up to 10% and involves removal of the distal stomach, duodenum and pancreatic head with anastomosis of stomach remnant, CBD and pancreatic tail onto the jejunum (Fig. 4). Unfortunately, pancreatic cancer often presents late and only 10% or so of patients undergo curative surgery.

Careful preoperative assessment is essential to prevent inappropriate surgery, and abdominal CT and laparoscopy are both useful. Surgery may also be useful for palliation if duodenal invasion has caused gastric outlet obstruction, when a gastro-jejunostomy can be performed. Chemotherapy has a very poor response rate, of the order of less than 10%. Consequently, the majority of patients require palliation for their jaundice and this is normally achieved endoscopically with stent placement. Full liaison with the palliative care team is required to maintain good pain control and to look after other aspects of palliative care.

The outlook is bleak with mean survival in the order of 3–6 months and the 1-year survival 8%.

CHOLANGIOCARCINOMA

Tumours of the biliary tree are almost invariably adenocarcinomas, which may occur anywhere along the biliary system, although two-thirds occur in the upper CBD. When the tumour is situated at the bifurcation of the left and right hepatic ducts, it is often termed a Klatskin tumour and can obstruct any one of the three ducts alone or in combination.

Tumours can be of a papillary or scirrhous form, and present in a similar way to carcinoma of the head of the pancreas with obstructive jaundice and weight loss.

There is probably an increased incidence of cholangiocarcinoma among patients with cholelithiasis (as the risk of cholangiocarcinoma appears to fall following cholecystectomy) but a stronger association exists with primary sclerosing cholangitis (PSC) and even long-standing ulcerative colitis in the absence of PSC may be associated with the development of cholangiocarcinoma. Chronic parasitisa-

tion by *Clonorchis sinensis* and possibly *Ascaris lumbricoides* leads to a rise in the incidence of cholangiocarcinoma in the Far East, where it accounts for 20% of primary liver tumours. Congenital cystic dilatation of the biliary tree also predisposes to cholangiocarcinoma.

Blood tests will show the usual picture for obstructive jaundice, but the alkaline phosphatase may be disproportionately raised.

Imaging in the patient with obstructive jaundice may give a clue that the aetiology is cholangiocarcinoma if, for example, dilated intrahepatic ducts are seen with a normal CBD. If the entire biliary tree is dilated down to the duodenum without visualisation of a pancreatic mass, this finding raises the possibility of a low cholangiocarcinoma or an ampullary tumour.

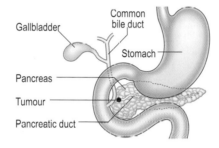

Before surgery

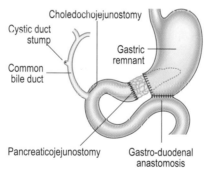

Whipple's operation

Fig. 4 **Whipple's operation.**

Diagnosis is usually made at ERCP when a papillary tumour or stricture is seen within the biliary system (Fig. 5). Confirmation can be with brush cytology or biopsy. Placement of an endoprosthesis is usually performed at the time. The diagnosis, like that of pancreatic cancer, is often made late and the condition is usually inoperable. Good palliation is normally possible by stenting. In the small proportion of patients that are operable only 5% will survive 5 years.

TUMOURS OF THE AMPULLA OF VATER

Occasionally, patients present with obstructive jaundice and at the time of ERCP are shown to have an ampullary tumour. These can be benign adenomas or, probably later in the history of the same lesion, can become neoplastic. They tend to present early because jaundice develops early, are slow growing and tend to do well following surgery. However, they often present in the aged patient and owing to anaesthetic risk are deemed inoperable.

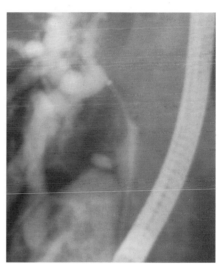

Fig. 5 **ERCP of cholangiocarcinoma showing a stricture in the mid common bile duct.**

Obstructive jaundice

- The development of obstructive jaundice with little or no pain, but with weight loss, in an elderly patient is most likely due to carcinoma of the head of the pancreas.
- Severe right upper quadrant pain associated with obstructive jaundice suggests stones.
- Ultrasound scanning is the method of choice for differentiating between a cholestatic jaundice and an obstructive jaundice.
- ERCP is the method of choice for helping to make a diagnosis and to palliate with stent placement.
- Patients usually present late in the illness and mean survival is 3–6 months.
- Cholangiocarcinoma is a more unusual cause of malignant obstruction, but it too is often inoperable and best treated with palliative stent placement.

TUMOURS AND ABSCESSES OF THE LIVER

TUMOURS

A common situation for clinicians to find themselves in is one in which a patient being investigated for non-specific symptoms such as weight loss or abdominal pain is demonstrated to have a mass or multiple lesions within the liver. These are commonly due to metastatic cancer, but not always, and the clinician must not assume that this is the case until it has been proven.

HISTORY AND EXAMINATION

A history must include age, sex and past medical history, systemic symptoms such as weight loss or pain and any other associated changes to the patient's normal well-being, such as a mass, change in bowel habit or bleeding.

The common sources for metastatic tumour in the liver are listed in Figure 1 and the history must include symptoms that may be associated with these organs. Examination may demonstrate a characteristically enlarged liver, which has an irregular surface. Breast examination is essential, as even small previously missed breast cancers can result in metastatic disease. Abdominal examination may reveal a mass or evidence of intestinal obstruction. Auscultation over the liver may demonstrate a vascular hum. In Asia and Africa hepatocellular carcinoma (HCC) is more common than metastatic tumours, because of the high prevalence of hepatitis B virus. Cirrhosis, induced by hepatitis B and C, alcohol, or iron overload all predispose to the development of HCC, and screening for this may be undertaken

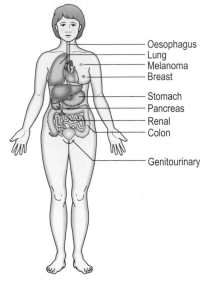

Fig. 1 **Sources of cancers that commonly metastasise to the liver.**

- Oesophagus
- Lung
- Melanoma
- Breast
- Stomach
- Pancreas
- Renal
- Colon
- Genitourinary

in these conditions. HCC may be found incidentally at post-mortem in up to 50% of patients with cirrhosis.

INVESTIGATIONS

Ultrasound scanning is the usual first investigation which may demonstrate discrete single or multiple lesions. The ultrasonographer may be confident that the lesions are due to tumours but this must not be relied upon, as focal nodular hyperplasia or discrete areas of fatty change can mislead the radiologist (Fig. 2).

CT scanning with contrast is often the next investigation which demonstrates low density lesions with ring enhancement following contrast injection (Fig. 3).

Blood test tests usually show an ele-

vated alkaline phosphatase and gamma glutamyl transpeptidase (GGT), and specific markers, such as carcinoembryonic antigen (CEA) in colonic cancer and α-fetoprotein (α-FP) in HCC, may be raised.

Biopsy is almost always necessary. The only exception would be in patients who are terminally ill, where the likelihood of intervention having a significant impact on survival is negligible. In all other cases, biopsy should be undertaken either under ultrasound guidance if a lesion is focal or as a blind percutaneous biopsy in more diffuse disease.

SECONDARY TUMOURS OF THE LIVER

Up until the last few years, a demonstration of hepatic metastases was an indication to institute palliative care and no consideration was given to active treatment. However, advances in chemotherapy and surgical resection have lead to a change in that approach. Some metastatic breast cancers respond quite well to chemotherapy, as may carcinoid tumours. Surgical resection of solitary hepatic metastases from colonic cancer can be undertaken and may even be curative. Multiple hepatic metastases or evidence of extrahepatic spread make this impossible.

There is often a dilemma regarding whether or not further investigation should be undertaken to identify the primary site, if the metastases are the first abnormality to be demonstrated. In advanced disease this is usually unnecessary, but an abdominal CT scan to demonstrate pancreatic and pelvic

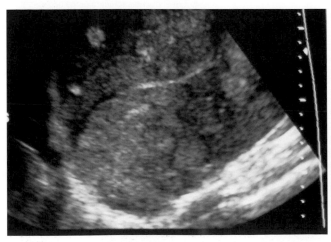

Fig. 2 **US scan of hepatic metastases.**

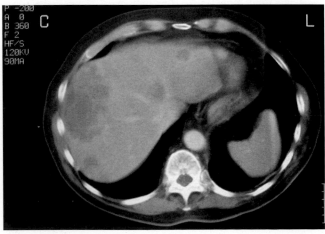

Fig. 3 **CT scan with contrast of hepatic metastases.**

lesions, and upper and lower GI endoscopy are most likely to yield a result if investigation is felt to be appropriate.

PRIMARY TUMOURS OF THE LIVER

Hepatocellular carcinoma (HCC) usually presents in patients with pre-existing liver disease. There may be a general deterioration in a patient's well-being, a fall in weight, decompensation with encephalopathy and ascites in a previously stable patient, or a lesion may be detected following screening. HCC is usually nodular (Fig. 4); although a diffuse infiltrative type is seen, which may be more difficult to detect radiologically. α-FP is a marker produced by 90% of HCC, but may be normal in small lesions. Values of > 400 ng/ml are indicative of HCC, although lesser elevations are seen in benign liver disease.

A rare HCC variant is the fibrolamellar type which presents in the young, with a large lesion usually in the absence of pre-existing liver disease. Tumours most commonly occur in the left lobe of the liver, tend not to produce α-FP and may be amenable to resection.

Less than a quarter of HCCs are resectable at diagnosis and 5-year survival rates are around 30%. Decompensated liver disease, invasion of the inferior vena cava, the portal vein or hepatic veins, extrahepatic spread or bilobar extension of HCC render it inoperable. Angiography is required preoperatively for assessment.

There is no effective alternative to surgery but injection of lesions with alcohol or embolisation may debulk large tumours.

Hepatic adenomas are tumours that affect women who have had the oral contraceptive pill (OCP) with high oestrogen content. This was particularly the case in the 1960s and as the oestrogen content of the OCP has fallen, so the incidence of this tumour has fallen. It presents as a well-demarcated large tumour, often with a palpable mass. Haemorrhage into the tumour causing pain may occur, or the tumour may rupture causing a haemoperitoneum. The OCP should be discontinued and, because of a risk of malignant transformation, surgical resection should be undertaken if possible.

Hepatic cysts are common, occurring in 2.5% of the population, but are usually asymptomatic. Ultrasound is the preferred method of detection and only rarely is aspiration necessary if the lesion is producing a mass effect. Hepatic cystadenomas are thick walled, with septa. They have a risk of malignant transformation and should be removed if possible.

Focal nodular hyperplasia is a rare benign tumour that most frequently affects women. It is non-encapsulated and is thought to develop around an area of arterial malformation. There does not appear to be a risk of bleeding or malignant transformation and the tumour can be left alone.

HEPATIC ABSCESS

These can be divided into pyogenic and amoebic, and differ widely in their clinical features. Patients with pyogenic liver abscess are usually middle-aged or older and have features of right upper quadrant pain, fever and weight loss. The usual source of the infection is intra-abdominal sepsis and there may be a preceding history suggestive of this, such as diverticular or biliary disease. Blood tests show a leucocytosis and blood cultures may be positive. Blood tests may show a normochromic normocytic anaemia, raised ESR and CRP. LFTs may show a rise in alkaline phosphatase and GGT, with modest changes in the aminotransferases. Ultrasound and CT are used to demonstrate the lesions and, if large enough, should be aspirated and drained. The commonest site to be affected is the right lobe of the liver, which is the area of highest portal blood flow. If abscesses are multiple, a biliary source of sepsis is more likely. Antibiotics with or without drainage may be necessary. A cephalosporin for Grams negative organisms, metronidazole for anaerobes and ampicillin for enterococci should be considered and adjusted in response to available cultures.

The biliary tree, and intra-abdominal diseases such as diverticulitis, Crohn's disease, ulcerative colitis and colon cancer may be complicated by liver abscess, and the GI tract should be investigated following recovery from the liver abscess.

Amoebic abscess is caused by *Entamoeba histolytica*, and follows travel to endemic areas. Symptoms are similar to those for a pyogenic abscess and blood tests are not discriminatory. Amoebic abscesses are often solitary and large and located in the right lobe of the liver. Serological testing is usually positive. If a pyogenic abscess is suspected, or rupture appears imminent, drainage should be undertaken. Otherwise metronidazole is the antibiotic of choice.

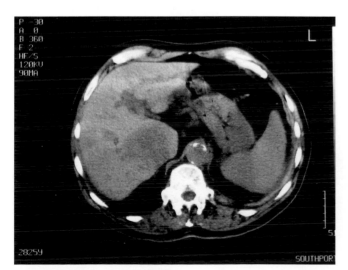

Fig. 4 **Hepatocellular carcinoma on CT.**

Tumours of the liver

- Metastatic disease of the liver is the commonest type of liver cancer in the Western world, but primary hepatocellular carcinoma is the commonest worldwide.
- Pre-existing cirrhosis due to chronic viral hepatitis, alcohol or iron overload predisposes to the development of HCC.
- Radiological suggestion of metastatic disease is insufficient to confirm the diagnosis and histology is required.
- Treatment for metastatic disease should be considered for all patients.
- Seeking the primary source in metastatic disease can be performed with abdominal and pelvic CT, and upper and lower endoscopy.

ACUTE HEPATITIS

Often, patients have an episode of acute hepatitis that is asymptomatic, but if present, symptoms include a feeling of general disability for a few days associated a with a mild temperature and generalized ache. When caused by a virus, there may be an episode of cholestasis with pale stools and dark urine which precedes the icteric phase. Patients become jaundiced and stools start to return to normal. Patients are often anorectic and there may be a feeling of nausea with a degree of tenderness over the liver. Examination reveals a generally well individual, who is jaundiced and without features of chronic liver disease.

The importance of taking a thorough history cannot be overemphasized. History of recent travel, injections, blood transfusions, ingestion of foods such as shellfish, use of recreational drugs both injected and those taken by alternative routes, all medications both prescribed and over-the-counter preparations for the last 3 months, and sexual activity, particularly homosexual contact, should be enquired about.

Early on in the illness, the alkaline phosphatase level may be elevated but the most marked feature is a rise in the serum aminotransferase concentrations with values often in the thousands. Serum bilirubin levels vary with the severity of the attack. Changes in the prothrombin time are usually absent or at most minor, except in the small proportion of patients who go on to develop fulminant hepatic failure.

Many drugs may produce this hepatitic picture but a number produce a pattern of cholestasis with elevation in the bilirubin, alkaline phosphatase and gamma glutamyl transpeptidase (GGT), without particular changes in the aminotransferases.

Blood should be drawn for viral studies and a monospot for glandular fever, which will allow confirmation of diagnosis at a later date, although this has little bearing on the acute management. All non-essential drugs should be discontinued, and patients should be encouraged to rest and may prefer a low fat diet. Alcohol should be avoided.

The usual clinical course is of a gradual resolution of the jaundice and general improvement in patient well-being. Complete recovery, however, may take some months, and patients should be warned of this. It is best to advise abstinence from alcohol for this period. If the episode is thought to be due to a drug reaction, then this agent must be avoided life-long. Depending on the virus, the episode may be followed by complete recovery or, in the case of hepatitis B and C, may develop into chronic hepatitis.

Occasionally, particularly following hepatitis A infection, patients have a prolonged cholestatic phase or have a minor relapse prior to complete resolution.

VIRUS-INDUCED ACUTE HEPATITIS

Hepatitis (HAV)

HAV is an RNA virus that is distributed worldwide and causes an acute hepatitis, particularly in children. It is transmitted by the faecal–oral route, usually with person-to-person contact, has an incubation period of 2–6 weeks and produces a typical hepatitis which may be subclinical (Fig. 1). The majority of children from underdeveloped countries have antibodies to HAV, but with improved sanitation, juvenile exposure is becoming less common in the West.

Diagnosis is made by detecting specific IgM antibody to HAV, which appears early in the infection and persists for 3–6 months.

Prevention is achieved by improving water supplies and sanitation, and a live vaccine is available for travellers to areas where HAV is prevalent.

The vast majority recover completely and HAV does not result in chronic liver disease.

Hepatitis E virus (HEV)

HEV is an RNA virus which, like HAV, is transmitted by the faecal–oral route and is related to poor sanitary conditions. It causes a similar clinical picture to that of HAV with an acute hepatitis which usually results in complete recovery. It is particularly prevalent in India and the Far East and does not result in chronic hepatitis, but may induce fulminant hepatic failure, particularly in pregnant women.

Infectious mononucleosis

Caused by the Epstein–Barr virus (EBV), infectious mononucleosis most commonly presents in teenagers, with typical features of a mild hepatitis often with a sore throat and submandibular lymphadenopathy. Up to a third may have a cholestatic pattern. Recovery is usually complete without sequelae, but fulminant hepatic failure may ensue, particularly in adults. Diagnosis is made with the detection of IgM antibodies to EBV and the monospot reaction is usually positive.

Table 1 **Causes of fulminant hepatic failure**

Drugs
Paracetamol
Halothane
Antidepressants
Non-steroidal anti-inflammatory drugs
Antituberculous drugs
'Ecstasy' (MDMA)
Carbon tetrachloride
Mushroom poisoning (*Amanita phalloides*)

Viruses
Hepatitis A (rare complication but represents 20% of FHF cases in developed countries)
Hepatitis B (most commonly associated agent worldwide)
Delta virus infection (in association with hepatitis B)
Hepatitis E (particularly pregnant women in Asia)
Hepatitis G (some reports of causing FHF in Japan)
Herpes simplex virus
Epstein–Barr virus

Pre-existing liver diseases that may present with FHF
Wilson's disease
Fatty liver of pregnancy
Liver ischaemia
Acute Budd–Chiari syndrome

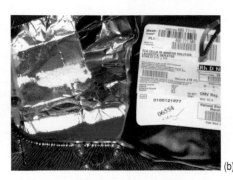

(a)   (b)

Fig. 1 **Source of faecal and oral transmission of hepatitis A (a) and parenteral sources of hepatitis B and C (b).**

Other viruses

Coxsackie B virus, cytomegalovirus (CMV) and paramyxoma viruses may all cause an acute hepatitis. Hepatitis B, hepatitis C and hepatitis D cause an acute hepatitis, but can also cause chronic hepatitis and are considered on page 102.

FULMINANT HEPATIC FAILURE

Fulminant hepatic failure develops when there has been a severe acute insult to the liver. There are a number of causes (Table 1) but in the UK the principal cause is paracetamol (acetaminophen) overdose. The important clinical features are jaundice, followed by the development of hepatic encephalopathy. The clinical presentation has been divided into 1) hyperacute, where encephalopathy develops within 7 days of the onset of jaundice; 2) acute, where the jaundice-to-encephalopathy period is between 8 and 28 days; 3) subacute where encephalopathy develops up to 26 weeks after the appearance of jaundice. This classification has important prognostic implications because the hyperacute group have the best outlook and their hepatic failure is most often due to paracetamol overdose.

Investigations must include 1) FBC to show evidence of an acute GI bleed or a low platelet count owing to consumption; 2) biochemistry to assess renal function; 3) LFTs' which characteristically show markedly elevated aminotransferases and the prothrombin time, which reflects severity.

To aid in diagnosing the cause of the hepatic failure, blood should be taken for estimation of paracetamol levels and detection of hepatitis A IgM and hepatitis B IgM anticore. Serum should be checked for anti-delta IgM if there has been a previous hepatitis B infection. Blood and urine should be cultured, arterial blood gases assessed, and the liver scanned by ultrasound.

Subsequent needle liver biopsy may be necessary. Severe hepatic damage results in a number of important consequences, such as the failure of clearance of gut endotoxin, with subsequent activation of macrophages and cytokine release, resulting in circulatory changes, tissue hypoxia, and finally multi-organ failure.

Management of these severely ill patients requires intensive care monitoring. Sepsis is a high risk and should be treated early and aggressively; patients may need intubation to protect their airway if in Grade 3/4 encephalopathy. Cerebral oedema, renal failure, circulatory dysfunction, coagulopathy and hypoglycaemia are all complications that may ensue.

Several specific treatment measures are sometimes necessary and include *N*-acetylcysteine if there is doubt about previous paracetamol overdose, forced diuresis in mushroom poisoning and acyclovir for herpes simplex virus infection.

In patients who fail to improve, liver transplantation must be considered, and the decision is based on the patient's age, the aetiology, time between onset of jaundice and encephalopathy and prothrombin time. Intercurrent bacterial infection is the commonest contraindication for liver transplantation and timing of the transplant is extremely difficult — patients should not receive a transplant too early when there is still a chance of spontaneous recovery or too late when the patient is terminally ill.

A number of alternatives to transplantation are being developed and include artificial liver support (an extracorporeal cartridges containing hepatocyte cell lines which may allow recovery or time for a liver to become available), and auxiliary liver transplants which are removed following recovery, obviating the need for long-term immunosuppression.

The prognosis is gloomy, with 36% surviving from the hyperacute group and just 7% surviving from the acute fulminant hepatic failure group.

THE LIVER AND INFECTION

It is common for there to be minor derangement in LFTs during any severe systemic infection, with rises in alkaline phosphatase, aminotransferases and GGT. If the source of infection is not clear, then occasionally the liver or biliary tract is considered as the potential source. Cholangitis should be considered, particularly in the presence of rigors. Ultrasound is generally poor at visualising CBD stones, and ERCP should be performed to exclude cholangitis.

Leptospirosis (Weil's disease)

This is an uncommon systemic infection caused by Leptospira icterohaemorrhagiae, an organism excreted in the urine of infected rats and which can remain in drains and canals for months. The illness most commonly occurs in people who have worked in drains. It is characterised by fever, abdominal and muscular pain. The central nervous system can be affected with headache and meningism. There may be a haemorrhagic tendency, and jaundice develops. Albuminuria and renal failure can develop subsequently. In the first week, spirochaetes may be found in the blood but beyond this serology is necessary to confirm the diagnosis. Treatment is with penicillin.

Peri-hepatitis

This is a rare condition caused by chlamydia which are thought to travel across the peritoneal cavity to the liver capsule from the female genital tract. It is characterised by right upper quadrant peritonsim in a young womn, and mild derangement of LFTs. Chlamydial serology may be positive but is non specific. 'Violin string' adhesions occur between liver capsule and adjacent structures which are seen at laparoscopy. Treatment is with tetracycline.

Acute hepatitis

- Acute hepatitis is often subclinical and complete spontaneous recovery usually occurs.
- Jaundice associated with a high transaminase level may follow a period of cholestasis.
- Hepatitis A virus does not cause a chronic hepatitis but may, rarely, result in fulminant hepatic failure.
- Fulminant hepatic failure is characterized by encephalopathy and jaundice.
- Fulminant hepatic failure requires close supportive management and early contact with a liver transplant unit.

DRUGS AND THE LIVER

Drug-induced liver disease accounts for up to 5% of hospital admissions for jaundice, and up to 20% of cases of fulminant hepatic failure. Drugs may produce liver damage predictably, in a dose-related fashion, such as paracetamol, or in an idiosyncratic reaction that is dose independent – and which occurs with a wide variety of drugs; indeed, a drug reaction should be considered in all patients who have taken any medication and who develop liver changes. Non-prescribed drugs should always be considered and enquired about, as recreational drugs such as cocaine and 'Ecstasy' (MDMA) may also induce liver injury.

Reactions can occur anything from a few days up to 3 months after ingestion, making a thorough drug history (with reference to the primary care practitioner if necessary) essential. The clinical pattern may be of an acute hepatitis with hepatocellular damage or of a cholestatic picture with pale stools, dark urine, itch.

The differential diagnosis includes acute liver injury due to viruses, toxins, immune hepatitis, and acute presentations of conditions such as Wilson's disease. In all cases, the drug needs to be withdrawn and the patient monitored for progression of liver damage. The majority undergo recovery without specific measures. For paracetamol, there is an antidote which should be given and is dealt with in the following section. Mild attacks require the exclusion of other causes and monitoring of a patient's progress with liver function tests including prothrombin time. Liver biopsy may be necessary if the diagnosis is in doubt or the patient is deteriorating.

DRUGS CAUSING AN ACUTE HEPATITIS

Paracetamol (acetaminophen)

Unfortunately, paracetamol is the commonest drug to cause liver damage and this is almost always as a result of deliberate overdose. It causes a predictable toxic effect in the liver and is the cause in over half of all cases referred to liver units with fulminant hepatic failure. In the UK, paracetamol-induced liver injury is responsible for 500 deaths annually. Other European countries are less troubled by paracetamol overdose, such as France where under 150 deaths occur per annum and this may be as a result of smaller pack size availability. Allowing over-the-counter purchase in only small pack numbers has been introduced in Britain and early figures suggest a fall in impulsive overdoses.

Paracetamol metabolism is well understood (Fig. 1). When the normal route is saturated, more N-acetyl-p-benzoquinone imine (NAPQI) is produced, which depletes glutathione stores and results in toxic injury. Glutathione is one of the major liver antioxidants and may be depleted under certain circumstances such as pre-existing liver disease or alcohol abuse. Enzyme inducers such as phenytoin may also increase patient susceptibility to paracetamol damage. Normally, doses in excess of 14 g are necessary to induce hepatocyte damage but in the above circumstances as little as 6 g may be all that is required.

Patients normally present to hospital admitting that they have taken an overdose and requesting help. The history should ascertain whether other drugs have been taken or if paracetamol was taken with alcohol or if there may be pre-existing liver disease. Blood is drawn for baseline studies including LFTs, a prothrombin time and for an estimate of the serum paracetamol concentration. A nomogram has been developed (Fig. 2) to determine who should be treated with the antidote and takes account of high-risk groups. The treatment is understandable when the mechanism by which paracetamol causes liver damage is understood and is aimed at replacing hepatic glutathione stores either with oral methionine or with intravenous N-acetyl cysteine (Table 2). To get an accurate estimate of serum concentration, 4 hours should have elapsed following the overdose, but in cases where there is a high likelihood of significant overdose, treatment should be initiated immediately and discontinued if serum concentrations later turn out to be below those necessary for treatment. Even in patients presenting late after paracetamol overdose, low-dose infusion of N-acetyl cysteine is helpful. Patients who present late often develop significant liver damage, and a prothrombin time of > 24 seconds at 24 hours following overdose represents severe disease. A high proportion of these individuals will develop fulminant hepatic failure, and a proportion will subsequently die.

Halothane

Halothane toxicity is a rare idiosyncratic reaction which occurs in 1:30 000 anaesthetic cases. It occurs particularly in those patients who are re-exposed to halothane within a month or in those with a previous reaction. Guidelines encouraging anaesthetists to avoid these circumstances have reduced this complication.

Isoniazid

This may occur 4–6 months after introduction, and presents with non-specific flu-like symptoms and a rise in the transaminases. A mild rise in the transaminases occurs in up to 20% of patients on isoniazid and often settles spontaneously. Older patients, co-treatment with rifampicin, previous liver disease or alcohol abuse increase the risk of toxicity. Paracetamol toxicity is increased, owing to enzyme induction by isoniazid.

Table 1 **Patterns of drug-induced liver damage**

	ALT	AP	ALT:AP ratio
Hepatocellular injury	> 2×	Normal	> 5
Cholestasis	Normal	> 2×	< 2
Mixed pattern	> 2	> 2	2–5

ALT = alanine aminotransferase; AP = alkaline phosphatase

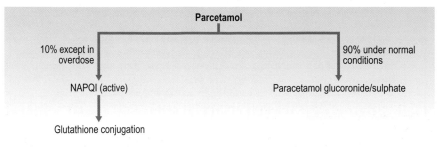

Fig. 1 **Paracetamol metabolism.**

DRUGS CAUSING A CHOLESTATIC PICTURE

Oestrogens

Oestrogens may induce cholestasis in patients, particularly those susceptible to cholestasis of pregnancy. Exogenous oestrogens given as a means of contraception are the usual source, but as doses used are lowering, it is becoming a less common complication.

Antibiotics

Penicillin derivatives such as flucloxacillin and augmentin may induce a cholestatic picture with jaundice, pale stools, dark urine and itch. This can occur several weeks after ingestion and usually resolves spontaneously; fatal cases have, however, been reported.

Chlorpromazine

This occurs in 1–2% of patients given the drug and usually within the first few weeks. A cholestatic picture develops with a peripheral eosinophilia. Resolution is usual following withdrawal of the drug, but may take many months.

DRUGS CAUSING A CHRONIC HEPATITIS

A number of drugs are recognised as having the potential of causing a chronic hepati-tis, similar to an autoimmune hepatitis. Differentiation can be difficult but patients improve following withdrawal of the drug. Nitrofurantoin and minocycline are both recognised as having this potential.

DRUGS CAUSING TUMOURS

Hepatic adenomas have been associated with oral contraceptive use, particularly of long duration and in older women.

DRUGS CAUSING A FATTY LIVER

Several drugs can cause a fatty liver, with a rise in aminotransferases that on occasion can lead to a full-blown hepatitis. Amiodarone, sodium valproate and verapamil are recognised to do this.

DRUGS CAUSING HEPATIC FIBROSIS

Methotrexate is now widely used in both rheumatology and dermatology, and to a lesser extent gastroenterology. Fibrosis develops following long-term use and seems less likely in patients receiving the drug for rheumatoid arthritis. It is recommended that patients should be monitored with LFTs whilst receiving the drug and should have it discontinued if the ALT rises by >3 x normal. LFTs do not accurately reflect the hepatic picture and following 1.5 g total of drug liver biopsy should be considered, and then repeated after a further 1.5 g. Significant fibrosis should lead to discontinuation.

DRUGS CAUSING GRANULOMATOUS DISEASE

When patients have had liver biopsies for abnormal LFTs (particularly a rise in alkaline phosphatase and GGT), granulomatous lesions are sometimes seen. The differential diagnosis of this is long and includes sarcoidosis, tuberculosis, berylliosis, brucellosis, a lymphoma or drugs. The list of drugs is long but includes allopurinol, chlorpromazine, diazepam, oral contraceptives, diltiazem and phenytoin.

As with all liver abnormalities, drugs should be considered and drug manufacturers or the Committee on Safety of Medicines (in the UK) consulted.

Table 2 **Treatment regimen for N-acetyl cysteine in paracetamol overdose**

- 150 mg/kg (patient weight) in 200 ml of 5% dextrose over 15 minutes; followed by
- 50 mg/kg in 500 ml of 5% dextrose over 4 hours; followed by
- 100 mg/kg in 1000 ml over 16 hours

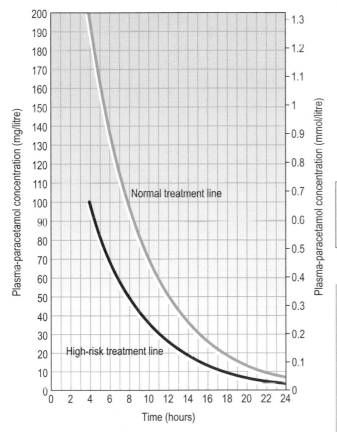

Fig. 2 **Paracetamol treatment nomogram.** Patients whose plasma–paracetamol concentrations are above the normal treatment line should be treated with acetyl cysteine by intravenous infusion. Patients on enzyme-inducing drugs (e.g. carbamazepine, phenobarbitone, phenytoin, rifampicin, and alcohol) or who are malnourished (e.g. in anorexia, in alcoholism, or those who are HIV-positive) should be treated if their plasma–paracetamol concentrations are above the high-risk treatment line. (Source: British National Formulary.)

Drugs and the liver

- Many drugs have the potential to cause liver damage, which may be predictable or idiosyncratic.
- All drugs, including prescribed, over-the-counter (non-prescription medication) and recreational (street) drugs should be considered.
- Drugs may cause a reaction months after ingestion.
- Paracetamol is the major cause of death due to drug-induced liver damage in Britain.
- Paracetamol-induced liver injury is caused by depletion of hepatic glutathione, which can be replaced by infusion of N-acetyl cysteine.

CHRONIC VIRAL HEPATITIS

Special mention is to be made of hepatitis B and C as they both have the capacity to cause chronic liver disease and are extremely widespread throughout the world, with perhaps 500 million carriers in total.

HEPATITIS B (HBV)

Epidemiology

HBV is a DNA virus which is transmitted parenterally or by intimate, often sexual, contact. Carrier rates vary from 0.1% in northern Europe and the USA, to 15% in the Far East, where transmission is usually perinatal and where infection of the newborn results in a chronic carrier state developing in 90% of children. Adults most commonly acquire the virus by sexual contact, particularly homosexual contact, intravenous drug abuse with shared needles, or following transfusion of infected blood. The converse of the situation in childhood occurs such that only 10% of adults will go on to become chronic carriers.

Serology

The virion has an outer surface antigen (HBsAg), which is produced in excess in the cytoplasm of the hepatocyte, and parts of which are released into the circulation. HBsAg is detectable 6 weeks following infection and non-clearance after 6 months denotes a carrier state. The core is within the surface protein and comprises a DNA polymerase, the DNA genome of HBV, and a core antigen (HBcAg) of which part is the e antigen (HBeAg) (Fig. 1). Detection of HBeAg suggests replication and high infectivity. IgM antibodies against HBcAg suggest recent infection and anti-HBs demonstrate immunity. HBV DNA is the most precise way of determining infectivity and is useful when considering treatment.

Clinical features

The majority of acute episodes are anicteric, and pass unnoticed. Rarely, acute hepatitis B results in fulminant hepatic failure, or a less severe episode of hepatitis – this usually results in viral clearance following recovery, as a brisk immune response is mounted by the host and clears the virus. Chronic carriage and therefore the risk of chronic liver disease develop in patients in whom the immune response is less effective, where either no response is mounted and patients become healthy carriers or where a weak response results in hepatocyte damage, but not viral clearance.

Patients are usually asymptomatic or may complain of fatigue. They may present with features of chronic liver disease or hepatocellular carcinoma which may complicate the condition. It is more usual to detect patients in the asymptomatic state, following screening health checks.

Treatment

If patients present late, with features of chronic liver disease, treatment is aimed at the complications such as varices and ascites from portal hypertension. Patients who present earlier may be candidates for treatment, but the majority of carriers will not go on to develop chronic liver disease. They are usually HBsAg, HBeAg and HBV DNA positive. Previously, treatment was with alpha interferon (IFN-α) for between 3 and 6 months – but response rates were in the order of 50% and drop-out due to the adverse effects of IFN-α (flu-like illness, neutropenia, alopecia, myalgia) were high. More recently, the newer agent lamivudine or 3TC (a reverse transcriptase inhibitor) has been used in patients with HBV and more advanced liver disease. Response rates are better, the agent is well tolerated and can be continued long term. Liver transplantation is an option for liver failure or poorly controlled complications of portal hypertension.

Effective hepatitis B vaccination is available and should be used in individuals involved in high-risk occupations or pastimes, such as health care workers, promiscuous adults, drug abusers, and near contacts and family of HBV patients who are not immune.

Affected individuals should be advised to avoid sharing intimate domestic items (toothbrushes, razors, etc.) and

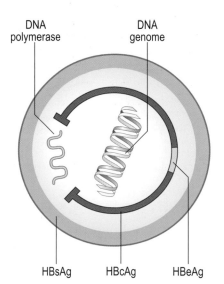

Fig. 1 **Structure of HBV.**

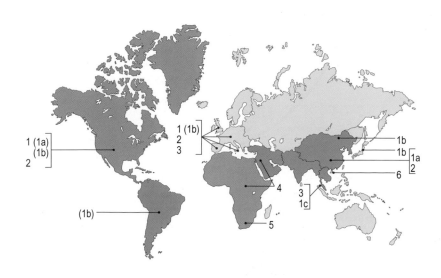

Fig. 2 **Geographical distribution of HCV genotypes and subtypes (from Brechot 1996).**

to practise safe sex with barrier contraception. Family members should be vaccinated.

Complications

A major concern is the development of hepatocellular carcinoma (HCC), particularly in males with longstanding disease, where ultrasound examination and serum α-fetoprotein concentrations should be checked regularly. Progression of liver disease is more marked in those who abuse alcohol. A deterioration may occur following an intercurrent hepatitis such as infection with hepatis A or delta virus (HDV). The latter only occurs in patients previously infected with HBV and requires HBsAg to replicate. It may result in an episode of active hepatitis and predisposes to more rapid progression of liver disease. Clearance of HBV results in the disappearance of HDV.

HEPATITIS C (HCV)

Epidemiology

HCV is an RNA virus discovered in 1989, which represents the majority of cases that were previously labelled non-A, non-B hepatitis. Worldwide prevalence varies, ranging from 1:1000 in northern Europe, to nearly 2% in the USA and up to 4% in Egypt.

Transmission is parenteral, via infected blood or blood products, and is particularly prevalent among current or former i.v. drug abusers who have shared needles, where infection rates in excess of 70% occur. Sexual and mother-to-infant transmission occur infrequently, although the prevalence is slightly higher amongst homosexual men (4%). Unlike HBV, the risk of becoming a chronic carrier following infection is high at around 80% and around a third of this group

may go on to develop serious chronic liver disease.

Serology

The first test available for HCV was an antibody test that relied on a single antigenic portion of HCV (c-100). This, unfortunately, had high sensitivity but low specificity. Later tests have used more than one antigen and have increased specificity. The later generation tests were introduced for screening of blood and blood products in the UK in 1991. However, there was a period, between the original test and the introduction of screening of donated blood, during which infected blood was used, and which has resulted in patients contracting HCV. Consequently, there has been a 'look-back' procedure, aimed at tracing individuals who received infected blood during that period. Following confirmation with enzyme-linked immu-nosorbent assay (ELISA), the polymerase chain reaction (PCR) is available to specifically detect the virus, and various genotypes, with various worldwide distributions, have been recognised (Fig. 2). This has implications for treatment, as genotype 1 (and 1b particularly) has a poor response rate in comparison to genotype 3.

Clinical features

Infection with HCV is usually anicteric and asymptomatic. It does not appear to cause fulminant hepatic failure. Individuals with HCV are usually asymptomatic but fatigue is a common symptom. Extrahepatic manifestations of HCV have been recognised and include arthritis, keratoconjunctivitis sicca and lichen planus. Autoantibodies such as cryoglobulinaemia and membranous glomerulonephritis occur in a small percentage of HCV patients. Cryoglobulins

are deposited in the glomeruli and in the extremities causing nephropathy and a vasculitis.

Treatment

Following a positive antibody test, viraemia should be confirmed with PCR and genotyping should be undertaken. Patients usually have a persistently elevated aminotransferase level, with an ALT of 100–200 U/l, and elevated GGT. These tests, however, do not reflect liver histology, and liver biopsy is essential to stage the disease. The history shows lymphoid aggregates in portal tracts, with sinusoidal infiltration by lymphocytes. Fatty change is common and fibrosis or cirrhosis may be present (Fig. 3).

Originally, treatment was with IFN-α, which was given for 6 months and had an initial response rate of 50%, but 50% of this group relapsed giving an overall response rate of only 25%. Recently, combination therapy has been introduced with ribavirin (a guanosine analogue), which has increased sustained response rates to around 50%, but this response rate ranges from 10% for genotype 1b to 70% for genotype 3.

The progression of liver disease is more likely in patients who also abuse alcohol, and abstinence is advised. Good responders are likely to have had the virus for a short period, have a low viral load, and be young and female.

A vaccine is not available.

Complications

As in HBV infection, there is an increased risk of developing HCC, with perhaps 1–2% of patients with HCV-induced cirrhosis developing this complication. About a third develop cirrhosis within 20 years of acquiring the virus, whilst many have inflammatory changes that do not progress to cirrhosis.

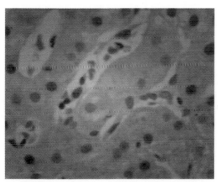

Fig. 3 **Sinusoidal lymphocytes and fatty change in HCV.**

Chronic viral hepatitis

- Hepatitis B virus and hepatitis C virus are the major causes of chronic hepatitis in the world.
- 90% of individuals infected with HBV as neonates will become carriers, whereas 90% of adults infected with HBV will clear the virus.
- Approximately 80% of individuals infected with HCV will become chronic carriers, of whom a majority will develop a degree of liver damage ranging from fatty liver to cirrhosis.
- Chronic HBV and HCV infection predispose patients to developing hepatocellular carcinoma.

AUTOIMMUNE HEPATITIS AND LIVER TRANSPLANTATION

AUTOIMMUNE HEPATITIS

Autoimmune hepatitis is a relatively uncommon condition that affects women much more commonly than men (4F : 1M) and whose aetiology is thought to be due to an inappropriate immune response to the liver. There appear to be two peaks of onset, the first in the third and fourth decades, in which the disease is often most aggressive, and a more indolent presentation in the fifth and sixth decades (Fig. 1).

As for other diseases considered to have an autoimmune basis, there are associations with HLA-B8-DR3 haplotype and particularly the DR3 and DR4 allotypes. There are associations with other autoimmune diseases such as thyroiditis, ulcerative colitis and Graves' disease.

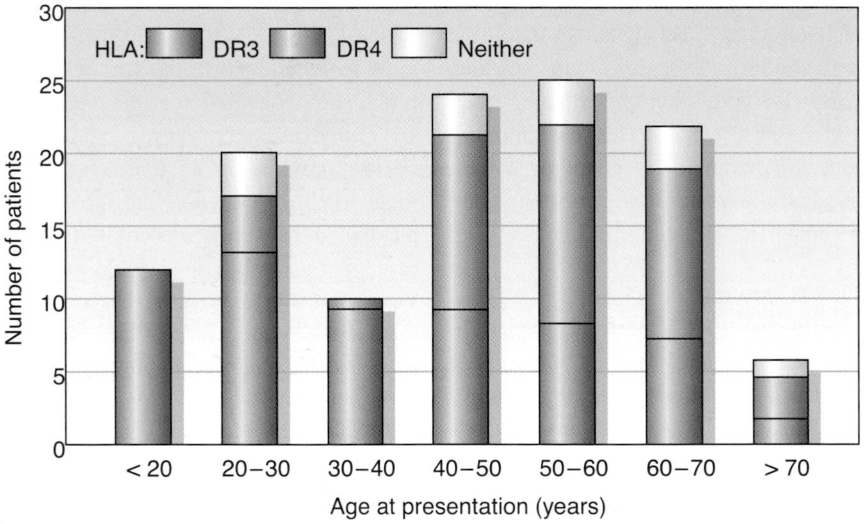

Fig. 1 **Distribution according to age at presentation and HLA-DR3 and -DR4 status of 118 adults with autoimmune hepatitis.**

PATHOLOGY

The characteristic histological picture in the liver is of a periportal hepatitis (interface hepatitis or piecemeal necrosis) with lymphocytes and plasma cells, without particular bile duct damage. The differential diagnosis particularly includes drug reactions, Wilson's disease and chronic viral hepatitis.

CLINICAL FEATURES

The presentation ranges between discovery of a mild chronic hepatitis following routine screening and a florid presentation with jaundice, a marked hepatitis and liver failure. Patients often describe a period of fatigue prior to the onset of jaundice and presumably have active hepatitis for months or years prior to becoming jaundiced. They are frequently amenorrhoeic and on examination have features of chronic liver disease and spider naevi. Blood tests confirm a hepatitis with aminotransferases usually more than 10 times normal, a raised bilirubin and clotting that is often deranged. There is a characteristic polyclonal rise in serum IgG concentrations and without this the diagnosis should be in doubt. There are specific autoantibody associations with antinuclear antibodies (ANA) – particularly the homogeneous pattern of staining (as in systemic lupus erythematosus), although other patterns of staining are seen. Smooth muscle antibodies (SMA) are present in two-thirds of patients but in low titre lack specificity, as they may be associated with other conditions such as primary biliary cirrhosis (PBC). The SMA react with a number of muscle components including actin and myosin – but this is probably not of clinical significance. Approximately 80% of patients with autoimmune hepatitis will present with ANA and/or SMA. Another autoantibody called the liver–kidney microsomal antibody (LKM-1) is present in a smaller number of patients, particularly younger women with more severe disease and without ANA or SMA. There may be an association between men with LKM-positive autoimmune hepatitis (AIH) and the hepatitis C virus, particularly in southern Europe, but the significance of this is unclear.

Various subtyping of AIH has been suggested depending on antibodies, with two broad groups described – type 1 where there is ANA/SMA positivity and type 2 where there is LKM-1 positivity, where the clinical course of the disease may be more aggressive and where there are more frequently other associated autoimmune diseases. It is important to exclude other potential causes of a hepatitis, and viral serology for hepatitis B and C should be performed, Wilson's disease should be excluded and a thorough drug history taken. Liver biopsy is necessary for diagnosis and staging, but occasionally has to be deferred following a presumptive diagnosis and initiation of treatment to allow the prothrombin time to normalise and the liver biopsy to be performed safely.

Around 20% of patients present with typical features as above, but without autoantibodies. They will have a hepatitic pattern of LFTs, an elevated serum IgG, and appropriate histological changes, and there may be associated autoimmune diseases. Treatment is as for antibody-positive AIH, and indeed a proportion of patients will become antibody-positive at a later stage.

TREATMENT

Immunosuppression with corticosteroids is the cornerstone of treatment, and patients are usually started on 30 mg of prednisolone, the condition brought under control and the dose gradually reduced. The dose can be reduced at 5 mg per week initially, but monitoring of the aminotransferases is necessary during this time to detect any rise, so that reduction can be stopped. It is now common to introduce azathioprine with the prednisolone in order to allow a lower maintenance dose of prednisolone and thus reduce the incidence of steroid-induced side-effects. Dosing is usually 50–100 mg azathioprine.

The majority of patients demonstrate improvement in the liver parameters over the first few weeks of treatment. Two-thirds achieve clinical remission within 3 years of treatment, and patients who do not have cirrhosis at presentation have a 10-year life expectancy that exceeds 90%, whilst in those with cirrhosis this figure is reduced to 65%.

Complications of steroid usage are common and where possible treated – such as in steroid-induced bone disease. Treatment is usually lifelong as discontinuation of therapy, even after some years, may result in relapse which may be more difficult to control. Features of chronic liver disease such as portal hypertension or ascites should be sought and treated conventionally. Risk of development of hepatocellular carcinoma is increased in long-standing disease and should be detected with a significant rise in the level of α-fetoprotein (α-FP) in the blood, although there is often a mild rise at the time of diagnosis that falls following treatment.

Liver transplantation should be considered when conventional immunosuppression has failed to induce remission or where the complications of cirrhosis have developed and are not responding to conventional medical therapy.

LIVER TRANSPLANTATION

For the first 20 years after the original human liver transplant in 1963, the procedure was rarely performed and had a poor outlook, but with the introduction of more effective immunosuppression, such as cyclosporin originally and tacrolimus more recently, plus changes in surgical technique, the procedure has become widely performed and is now a recognised treatment modality for many severe liver diseases. Indications for transplantation can be broadly divided in two:

- those that require a transplant because of fulminant hepatic failure, usually owing to drugs such as paracetamol, or viruses
- those with chronic liver failure because of conditions such as PBC, alcoholic liver disease, and advanced chronic liver disease due to viruses (Table 1).

The indication for transplantation strongly affects outcome so that patients transplanted for acute liver failure have a 1-year survival of around 60%, whilst those transplanted for chronic stable liver disease such as PBC have a 1-year survival of 90%.

DONOR SELECTION

There is a general shortage of donor livers and to try to optimise the numbers available a coordinated programme is operative in the UK, with transplant coordinators visiting sites where donor organs may be available. Donors have usually suffered irreversible brain injury without there having been significant hypotension or anoxia, nor should there be other significant diseases such as diabetes or malignancy.

RECIPIENT SELECTION

Selection and timing are major difficulties for hepatologists. In fulminant hepatic failure, patients should not be moribund, but should not be operated upon when there is still a good chance of spontaneous recovery. Referral to a transplant centre should have occurred prior to the criteria in Table 2 having been met, as patients fulfilling any of these criteria have a > 80% mortality.

Selection of patients with chronic liver disease usually has the advantage of time, but again needs to be done before the patient has become terminally ill. PBC has a more defined progression and patients with a bilirubin of > 100 mmol/l, or evidence of decompensation such as uncontrollable ascites or bleeding oesophageal varices should be referred.

Livers are matched for size, and ABO compatibility. Following removal from the donor, they are transported cooled and perfused with University of Wisconsin solution to improve storage.

In the immediate postoperative period, problems with haemorrhage and portal vein or hepatic artery thrombosis are most common, in addition to problems relating to the recipient's general medical condition, such as cardiovascular and respiratory disease. 7–10 days after transplantation acute rejection can occur, which can be treated with high-dose steroids, whilst later on, chronic rejection with vanishing bile ducts at histology represents a more serious complication and can result in graft failure.

Immunosuppressive requirements often lessen with time, so that minimal treatment is often required in the long term.

Table 1 **Conditions that should be considered for transplantation**

Acute liver failure
Viruses disease
Drugs (paracetamol, isoniazid, halothane, etc.)
Metabolic liver diseases (Wilson's)
Chronic liver failure
Primary biliary cirrhosis
Primary sclerosing cholangitis
Alcoholic cirrhosis
Chronic immune hepatitis
Veno-occlusive disease (Budd–Chiari)
Congenital/metabolic
Biliary atresia
Haemochromatosis
Wilson's disease
Glycogen storage disease

Table 2 **Criteria for transplantation in fulminant hepatic failure**

Paracetamol induced
pH < 7.30
or
Prothrombin time of > 100 s and serum creatinine of >300 μmol/l in patients with grade III or IV encephalopathy
Non-paracetamol patients
Prothrombin time > 100 s (irrespective of grade of encephalopathy)
or
Any three of the following (irrespective of grade of encephalopathy):
Age < 10 or > 40 years
Aetiology non-A, non-B hepatitis, halothane or idiosyncratic drug reactions
Duration of jaundice before onset of encephalopathy of > 7 days
Prothrombin time > 50 s
Serum bilirubin > 300 μmol/l

Autoimmune hepatitis and liver transplantation

- Autoimmune hepatitis is four times more common in women than in men, and is most aggressive when it presents in the third and fourth decades.
- AIH can be associated with other autoimmune diseases.
- Important differential diagnoses include viral hepatitis, Wilson's disease and drug reactions.
- There is a rise in IgG, a positive anti-smooth-muscle antibody present in 60%, and antinuclear antibody and LKM-1 antibody may be present.
- Long-term immunosuppression is required with corticosteroids and often azathioprine.
- Liver transplantation should be considered for most patients with end-stage liver disease or acute fulminant hepatic failure, and transplant units should be contacted early regarding referral.

PREGNANCY AND LIVER DISEASE

There are some liver conditions that are specific to pregnancy, but it should not be forgotten that the usual array of liver disease that affects non-pregnant women may also affect those that are pregnant. Viral hepatitis, immune hepatitis, primary biliary cirrhosis, gallstones, and drug reactions may all present during pregnancy and should not be forgotten (Fig. 1).

When confronted with a pregnant woman who has developed abnormal liver function tests or become jaundice, start as usual with a thorough history including pre-existing conditions and drugs taken over the preceding 6 months (prescribed, over the counter and recreational). Examination may demonstrate features of chronic liver disease, but will often be normal. Initial investigations will include bloodtests – full blood count, liver function tests, virology including hepatitis A serology and monospot for infectious mononucleosis, autoantibodies for anti-smooth muscle antibodies and anti-mitochondrial antibodies. Liver ultrasound may demonstrate fatty liver, gallstones and an obstructed biliary system if present. Pre-existing liver disease may also worsen or become apparent during pregnancy, and usually requires continuation of particular treatments such as corticosteroids in autoimmune hepatitis, and penicillamine in Wilson's disease, with close monitoring.

However, pregnancies are unusual in women with cirrhosis. Oesophageal varices may be more likely to bleed during pregnancy and their treatment should be continued in the conventional manner.

NORMAL CHANGES IN PREGNANCY

The majority of LFTs remain unchanged during pregnancy but albumin may fall and the alkaline phosphatase (AP) often rises but does not exceed a four-fold increase. This is due to placental production and AP does not usually rise until the third trimester. The gamma glutamyl transpeptidase (GGT) should remain normal if the alkaline phosphatase is of placental origin.

CONDITIONS SPECIFIC TO PREGNANCY
First trimester / second trimester

Hyperemesis gravidarum
Severe vomiting during the first trimester can result in a modest rise in the bilirubin and alkaline phosphatase levels but severe liver damage is not a feature. The condition can recur in subsequent pregnancies.

Dubin–Johnson syndrome
This may present in pregnancy as oestrogens appear to aggravate it. There is a rise in conjugated bilirubin without other LFT changes. No specific treatment is required.

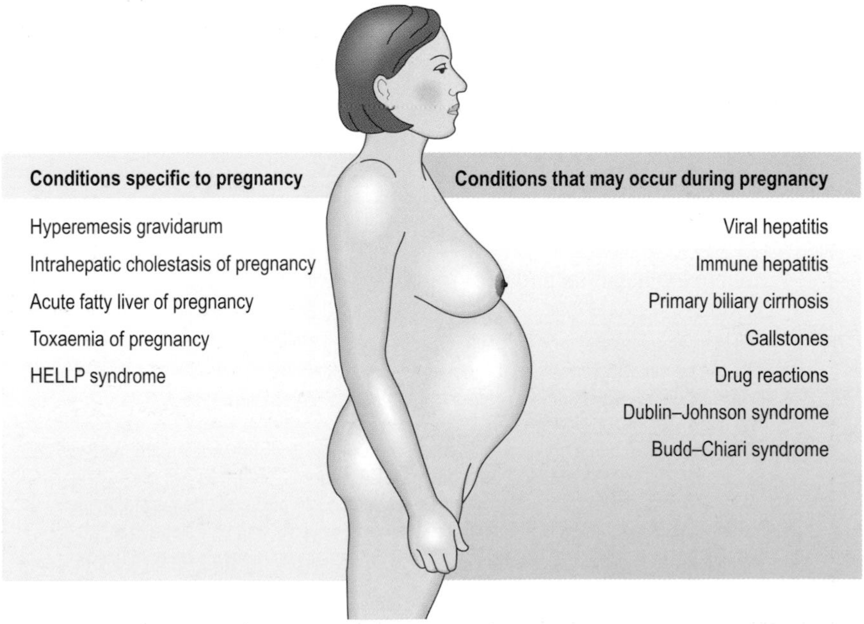

Third trimester
Cholestasis of pregnancy
Also known as intrahepatic cholestasis of pregnancy, benign recurrent cholestasis of pregnancy and pruritus gravidarum, this condition usually presents in the third trimester but may present earlier. It may be familial with mothers, sisters and daughters being affected, is often worse with multiple pregnancies and may recur with menstruation or oestrogen therapy after pregnancy, implying a hormonal aetiology. Its reported incidence ranges from 0.1% of pregnancies in most European countries to 10% in Chile.

The clinical features are typical for cholestasis, with pruritus, pale stools and dark urine. There is elevation in the conjugated bilirubin and alkaline phosphatase, and the prothrombin time is prolonged because of vitamin K malabsorption. There may be an association with HLA-BW16 and male relatives may also show a predisposition to cholestasis when given oestrogen. Liver biopsy is usually not necessary, but may show areas of cholestasis. Treatment is with cholestyramine for pruritus and parenteral vitamin K to correct clotting abnormalities. There are usually no long-term sequelae for the mother but postpartum haemorrhage may be more likely if the prothrombin time is not corrected. There is an increase in perinatal mortality. Differential diagnosis includes drug reactions and primary biliary cirrhosis. The patient should be warned that the condition may recur in subsequent pregnancies.

Acute fatty liver of pregnancy
This is a rare (1:13 000) complication of pregnancy which normally occurs in the last 8–9 weeks of gestation. The condition presents with nausea, vomiting and abdominal pain which is then followed in a few days by jaundice. Ascites develops in 50%. There are associations with male offspring, first pregnancies, hypertension and proteinuria. Jaundice is present without haemolysis and there is a moderate elevation in the aminotransferases. Platelet count falls, prothrombin time rises, hypoglycaemia is prominent, and there are rises in the serum uric acid and ammonia levels.

The important differential diagnoses are of a viral hepatitis or a drug reaction.

Conditions specific to pregnancy	Conditions that may occur during pregnancy
Hyperemesis gravidarum	Viral hepatitis
Intrahepatic cholestasis of pregnancy	Immune hepatitis
Acute fatty liver of pregnancy	Primary biliary cirrhosis
Toxaemia of pregnancy	Gallstones
HELLP syndrome	Drug reactions
	Dublin–Johnson syndrome
	Budd–Chiari syndrome

Fig. 1 **Pregnancy and liver disease.**

Previously, maternal mortality was as high as 80–90%. It is now considerably lower at ~ 10%, but there is still a high fetal mortality. Maternal death usually results from the complications of disseminated intravascular coagulation or renal failure. Patients need careful monitoring and if symptoms of nausea and vomiting are persisting or worsening, then the child should be delivered. Supportive care is then necessary for the mother during recovery.

Toxaemia of pregnancy

Usually occurring after the 20th week of gestation, toxaemia of pregnancy is characterised by hypertension, proteinuria and oedema. Changes in the aminotransferases and alkaline phosphatase may occur but are usually mild. If jaundice develops, this is usually associated with haemolysis and disseminated intravascular coagulation and denotes severe toxaemia.

HELLP syndrome (Haemolysis, Elevated Liver enzymes and Low Platelets)

This is probably a variant of toxaemia of pregnancy associated with disseminated intravascular coagulation.

Rarely, toxaemia can be complicated by hepatic haemorrhage or liver rupture. There is severe right upper quadrant pain associated with circulatory collapse. Ultrasound scanning will demonstrate the bleed. Mild cases can be treated supportively, whereas more severe cases may need surgery. There is an associated high mortality.

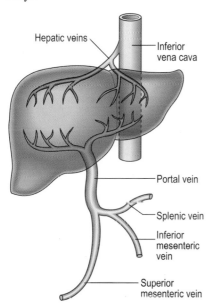

Fig. 2 **Portal and hepatic vein anatomy.**

Budd–Chiari syndrome

Budd–Chiari syndrome usually presents in the immediate postpartum period and is characterised by right upper quadrant pain, tender hepatomegaly and the sudden appearance of ascites. The ascitic fluid normally has a high protein content. There are modest changes in serum aminotransferases and alkaline phosphatase. A hepatic venogram shows the underlying problem of thrombosis in either hepatic veins or the inferior vena cava. There is sparing of the caudate lobe of the liver as this normally drains directly into the inferior vena cava. Anticoagulation is usually unhelpful but early thrombolytic therapy may help. The condition carries a poor prognosis.

Occasionally confusion exists between hepatic (Budd–Chiari) and portal vein thrombosis (Fig. 2). They produce quite different clinical pictures. Portal vein thrombosis occurs as a result of local sepsis, inflammatory bowel disease, pancreatitis or following splenectomy. Portal vein sepsis is common in India and accounts for a significant proportion of variceal bleeds. Hypercoagulable states such as protein C or S deficiency and factor V leiden may predispose to portal vein thrombosis. Clinically, the liver is of normal size and function. Splenomegaly is usual and patients often present with variceal haemorrhage. There are no features of chronic liver disease and clotting factors are normal. Ascites may be present and hepatic encephalopathy may develop following a GI bleed (due to the liver being bypassed by shunts).

The portal vein cannot be identified on Doppler and multiple small collateral vessels develop around the portal vein return-

ing to the liver. MR may demonstrate these changes.

The outlook is better than for portal hypertension due to chronic liver disease as liver function is generally normal. Bleeding varices are treated conventionally, but fundal varices can be a problem particularly in splenic vein thrombosis.

Viral hepatitis

Infection with hepatitis E virus is usually a self-limiting episode which is rarely associated with fulminant hepatic failure, but in pregnant women the frequency of development of this complication is up to 25% with a very high associated mortality. This has particularly been reported from India and the Middle East.

If the mother has an acute clinical episode associated with hepatitis B virus during the first trimester, neonatal transmission is very low. This rises through the second and third trimesters such that mothers who are acutely ill during the third trimester have a neonatal transmission rate of 70%. This rises further if the mother is acutely ill during the first 2 months after delivery, which is explained by the mother being particularly infectious during the incubation period, which occurs when the child is still in utero

Children born to HBV-positive mothers can have the risk of developing HBV reduced by 90% by early administration of hepatitis B immune globulin, given at birth and followed by HBV vaccination at 7 days, 1 month and 6 months.

HCV transmission from mother to baby occurs infrequently, and there is no evidence that transmission occurs following breast-feeding.

Pregnancy and liver disease

- Liver disease developing during pregnancy is not necessarily related to the pregnancy, and other causes of liver disease should not be forgotten.
- Intrahepatic cholestasis of pregnancy causes a cholestatic picture and tends to run a benign course.
- Acute fatty liver of pregnancy is a serious complication of pregnancy and carries a significant mortality.

NORMAL NUTRITION

DAILY REQUIREMENTS

Energy

The total daily energy expenditure (TEE) varies according to morphology, physical activity and illnesses such as sepsis or surgery. The resting metabolic rate (RMR) represents ~ 70% of TEE, the thermic effect of food ~ 15% and the thermic effect of physical activity ~ 15% of TEE (Fig. 1). The RMR depends on lean body mass, and may fall by 15% during starvation but rise by 20% during sepsis. Dietary energy supplied by fat ranges from 10% in poorer parts of Africa to 80% in more affluent societies. When artificially feeding patients, proportions can be adjusted, but approximately 30% of non-protein energy should come from lipid and 70% from carbohydrate. In patients with Crohn's disease, lower fat concentrations may be better tolerated.

Protein

Daily protein requirements depend on factors such as total caloric intake, protein quality, the patient's nutritional status, and 'metabolic conditions' such as illness or injury which may increase requirement from a mean of 0.75 g/kg/day to 1.5 g/kg/day. Requirement can be calculated using nitrogen balance where 6.25 g protein provides 1 g of nitrogen in the diet. Nitrogen loss can be measured in urine and stools. A negative nitrogen balance rapidly leads to protein loss from the liver and then muscle. The protein intake must contain the essential amino acids.

Carbohydrate

There are no obligatory dietary carbohydrate requirements but an average diet contains 400 g of digestible carbohydrate of which 60% is starch, 30% sucrose and 10% lactose. About 10–20 g of indigestible carbohydrates (fibre) is eaten per day.

Lipids

Dietary fat contains predominately triglycerides of 16–18 carbon length which may be saturated or unsaturated. Some fatty acids cannot be synthesised

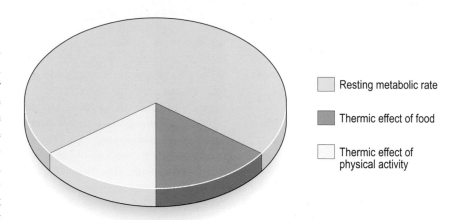

Fig. 1 **Constituent components of total energy expenditure of a well individual.**

Resting metabolic rate

Thermic effect of food

Thermic effect of physical activity

by the liver and are essential dietary components. Medium-chain triglycerides do not require bile to be absorbed and may be a useful dietary supplement in people with malabsorption.

Major minerals

Major minerals are those that require an intake of greater than 100 mg a day and include sodium, potassium, magnesium, calcium and phosphorus.

Trace elements

These are inorganic nutrients of which less than 100 mg a day are required and include iron, zinc, copper, chromium and iodine.

Vitamins

These are organic compounds that are required in small quantities (< 100 mg/day) and deficiency of which may lead to recognisable clinical syndromes (Table 1).

Table 1 **Vitamin requirements and findings in deficiency**

Micronutrient	RDA*	Deficiency
Fat-soluble vitamins		
Vitamin A	5000 IU	Follicular hyperkeratosis, night blindness, keratomalacia
Vitamin D	400 IU	Rickets, osteomalacia, muscle weakness
Vitamin E	10–15 IU	Haemolysis, neuropathy
Vitamin K	50–100 μcg	Prolonged prothrombin time, easy bruising
Water-soluble vitamins		
Vitamin C	60 mg	Scurvy – poor wound healing, perifollicular haemorrhage, gingivitis
Vitamin B_1 (thiamine)	1–1.5 mg	Dry beriberi – polyneuropathy, low temperature Wet beriberi – high-output cardiac failure Wernicke–Korsakoff syndrome – ataxia, nystagmus, confabulation, ophthalmoplegia
Vitamin B_2 (riboflavin)	1.1–1.8 mg	Seborrhoeic dermatitis, stomatitis, geographic tongue
Vitamin B_3 (niacin)	12–20 mg	Anorexia, lethargy, glossitis Pellagra – diarrhoea, dermatitis, dementia
Vitamin B_6 (pyridoxine)	1–2 mg	Peripheral neuritis, seborrhoeic dermatitis, stomatitis
Vitamin B_9 (folic acid)	400 μcg	Megaloblastic anaemia, glossitis, paraesthesiae
Vitamin B_{12}	3 μcg	Megaloblastic anaemia, dorsal column sensory loss
Major minerals		
Sodium	100–150 mmol	Hypovolaemia, weakness
Potassium	60–100 mmol	Weakness, paraesthesiae, arrhythmias
Magnesium	5–15 mmol	Weakness, twitching, arrhythmias
Calcium	5–15 mmol	Osteopenia, tetany, arrhythmias
Phosphorus	20–60 mmol	Weakness, fatigue, haemolysis
Trace elements		
Iron	1–1.5 mg	Microcytic hypochromic anaemia
Zinc	2.5–4 mg	Alopecia, diarrhoea, mental changes
Copper	0.3 mg	Anaemia, neutropenia, lethargy
Chromium	10–20 μcg	Glucose intolerance, peripheral neuropathy
* Recommended daily allowance		

ASSESSMENT

Reliably assessing a patient's nutritional status is surprisingly difficult, as there is no single measurement or calculation that will assess all patients. Consequently, deciding whether a patient is undernourished and requires nutritional support is a decision based upon knowledge of previous nutritional state, recent changes in dietary intake, current nutritional status and ongoing illness. Skinfold thickness and bioelectric impedance analysis allows estimates of subcutaneous fat stores, and assay of micronutrients such as red cell folate and ferritin can demonstrate specific nutritional deficiencies. Serum albumin falls upon starvation, but may also fall as part of an acute-phase reaction and is therefore a poor discriminator. In everyday clinical practice, documentation of height, weight (with comparison of previous weights to assess weight change) and clinical examination which assesses fat stores, taken in combination with the underlying disease, should allow a decision to be made as to whether nutritional supplementation should be given. Some conditions such as Crohn's disease may have specific benefits related to feeding and these patients will be fed as a treatment. Other patients with sepsis, inflammation, or malignancy will often benefit from nutritional supplementation.

Assessing overweight patients is a little easier and perhaps less critical. A body mass index can easily be calculated (weight in kg/(height in m)^2) and a normal value falls below 25 with the morbidly obese having an index of > 40.

NUTRITIONAL SUPPORT

Enteral feeding

Enteral feeding is the preferred option for patients who need nutritional support but are unable to manage this independently. The most common indication is following neurological events such as strokes, where the swallowing mechanism is either temporarily or permanently disrupted. Other indications include pre-radiotherapy or after surgery to the oropharynx or oesophagus, which will temporarily disrupt swallowing. The advent of fine-bore nasogastric tubes (Fig. 2), which are moderately well toler-

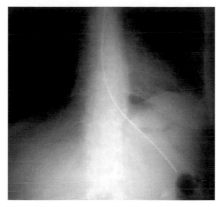

Fig. 2 **Fine-bore nasogastric tube into the stomach visible on upper right.**

ated by patients, means that nasogastric feeding can be maintained with reasonable comfort for up to 2–3 weeks. If feeding is required beyond this period, then it is usually best to place a percutaneous endoscopic gastrostomy (PEG) tube.

A selection of liquid feeds are available that vary in their caloric concentration, and fat, protein and carbohydrate concentrations. Feeds should be selected following discussion with a dietitian to determine each patient's requirements.

Complications that may occur with nasogastric feeding include inadvertent tracheal placement of the tube, and positioning must be confirmed either by acid aspiration or following X-ray. Aspiration may also occur with tubes appropriately placed within the stomach, particularly if feed is administered too quickly, or the patient is recumbent. If gastric emptying is impaired, a promotility agent may be helpful. Diarrhoea can develop, and dilution of feed and a slower infusion rate may help this problem. Other causes of diarrhoea such as pseudomembranous colitis and pancreatic insufficiency should not be forgotten.

Problems specific to PEG tubes may be related to their placement (which is dealt with on p. 16), and also include local sepsis, tube displacement or blockage, and leakage around the tube.

Parenteral feeding

As more is understood about the nutritional requirements of the ill patient, parenteral feeding is becoming more common. Feeding can be administered via a peripheral line but only feeds of low osmolality can be given, as phlebitis and thrombosis can otherwise develop. This is an acceptable route if feeding is for a short period of less than 7 days – longer periods require placement of a catheter into a central vein. The catheter must be placed with the strictest of sterile techniques so as to avoid the major complication of feeding via this route – namely line sepsis.

Feeds are individualised to the patients' requirements and are adjusted daily according to their biochemistry.

Problems related to this type of feeding include sepsis, pneumothorax, thrombosis, metabolic abnormalities, gastrointestinal mucosal atrophy and hepatic abnormalities.

WEIGHT LOSS

It is first important to confirm and quantify actual weight loss. Patients will frequently report that they have lost considerable amounts of weight but when details about previous weight are available patients have often overestimated their loss. As with any symptom where there is a very broad differential diagnosis' an ordered approach to diagnosis is required so that investigations can be focused. Usually within a history there are clues to direct the clinician, and specific enquiry should be made about

Table 2 **Causes of weight loss**

Inflammatory/infective
Inflammatory bowel disease
Abscesses
Bacterial endocarditis
Tuberculosis
AIDS
Neoplastic
Pancreatic cancer
Gastric cancer
Bowel cancer
Lung cancer
Disseminated cancer
Haematological malignancy
Metabolic/endocrine
Diabetes
Thyrotoxicosis
Addison's disease
Hypopituitarism
Malabsorption
Coeliac disease
Chronic pancreatitis
Disordered swallowing/ingestion
Achalasia
Gastric outflow obstruction
Psychiatric
Depression
Eating disorder – anorexia nervosa/bulimia
Chronic diseases
Chronic pulmonary disease
Chronic heart failure
Neurological disease
Motor neurone disease

intake, malabsorption, possible neoplastic disease, eating disorder and depression.

The possibilities are numerous (Table 2) so the clinician is often wary about making a diagnosis of depression for fear of missing another potentially fatal disease. If treatment is instituted for this condition, an open mind should always be kept because serious diseases can coexist with depression.

ANOREXIA NERVOSA

A devastating illness that predominately afflicts young females (95%), anorexia nervosa needs to be recognised and treated effectively. Patients often present to gastroenterologists for exclusion of other GI disorders, such as Crohn's disease or coeliac disease. The outlook is distressingly poor, with mortalities quoted in excess of 10%.

Clinical features include a fear of gaining weight and a refusal to maintain body weight at or above a minimally normal weight for age and height. There is often a disturbance of body image and undue influence of body weight or shape on self-evaluation. There is a lack of realisation of the seriousness of the low body weight. Amenorrhoea (absence of > 3 consecutive menstrual cycles), fine downy hair (lanugo), abnormal dentition and calluses on the dorsum of the hand when vomiting has been induced, may be seen on examination. Patients will often exercise unduly and manipulate their family, friends and physicians. Abuse of laxatives and diuretics may also be seen. Haematological abnormalities such as leucopenia and a normocytic anaemia can occur.

Management is usually psychological but medical input can be necessary in those of very low weight to prevent death and because psychological therapies are unlikely to be successful in the grossly underweight.

Bulimia nervosa is characterised by similar features to anorexia nervosa but there is binge eating with excessive intake associated with induced vomiting or laxative abuse.

WEIGHT GAIN

Occasionally, gastroenterologists are asked to review patients who feel that their weight increase is not solely due to their increased food intake or decreased exercise but feel that there may be an alternative explanation. Rarely, hypothyroidism and Cushing's disease may cause obesity and these can be excluded by demonstrating a normal thyroid-stimulating hormone, and dexamethasone suppression test. A wide range of medications can lead to weight gain (Table 3) and these should be sought in the history. Depression may lead to overeating and care should be taken in choosing the medical therapy for this, as some antidepressants encourage weight gain.

Extremely rarely, tumours or trauma that affect the hypothalamus can result in obesity as may a number of rare congenital syndromes.

The most useful parameter in an obese patient is the proportion of body fat, which can be determined by various methods including total body bioelectric impedance which is now readily performed. Waist–hip ratios are also useful, as an increase in this ratio (i.e. increased abdominal girth) correlates with an increase in complications such as ischaemic heart disease and stroke. Various definitions of obesity exist, including a weight of > 20% above ideal, or a body mass index (BMI = weight in kg/(height in m)^2) of > 27.3 in women and 27.8 in men, whilst morbid obesity can be defined as a BMI of > 40. The BMI has the advantage of ease of measurement and is widely used. Potential complications of obesity are listed in Table 4.

Treatment is usually with dietary modification, which should be long-term to achieve sustained slow weight loss. Orlistat is a pancreatic lipase inhibitor which can be used in conjunction with dietary restriction, but as with many treatments for obesity, the effects appear not to be sustained following discontinuation of therapy. Surgical therapy is rarely used and includes jejunoileal bypass which can be complicated by severe biochemical abnormalities and liver disease, and gastric restriction procedures such as banding gastroplasty.

Table 3 **Drugs that are associated with weight gain**

Hormonal/endocrine therapies
Corticosteroids
Hormone replacement therapy
Oral contraceptive pill
Sulphonylureas

Psychiatric medications
Amitriptyline
Citalopram (selective serotonin re-uptake inhibitor)
Chlorpromazine
Lithium

Table 4 **Complications of obesity**

Gastrointestinal
Gastro-oesophageal reflux
Gallstones (particularly following weight loss)
Liver abnormalities (fatty liver, fibrosis and cirrhosis)
Pancreatitis (gallstones and hypertriglyceridaemia)
Increased risk of colorectal cancer

Cardiovascular
Ischaemic heart disease
Hypertension
Stroke
Peripheral vascular disease

Hormonal
Maturity onset diabetes

Musculoskeletal
Osteoarthritis

Respiratory
Restricted respiration

Normal nutrition

- Resting metabolic rate uses 70% of total energy expenditure but this proportion can fall by 15% during starvation and rise by 20% during illness.
- Dietary protein requirements vary from 0.75 g/kg/day to 1.5 g/kg/day, depending on sepsis or illness.
- 6.25 g of dietary protein provides 1 g nitrogen.
- Body mass index is readily calculated in the clinic as weight in kg/(height in m)^2.
- Peripheral line TPN can be used for periods of feeding of less than 7 days; beyond this a central venous catheter should be placed for feeding.

INDEX